Leave No Nurse Behind: Nurses Working with disAbilities

Leave No Nurse Behind: Nurses Working with disAbilities

Donna Carol Maheady, ARNP, EdD

*Preface by Donna Cardillo, RN, MA, creator of **Career Alternatives for Nurses**™*

iUniverse, Inc.

New York Lincoln Shanghai

Leave No Nurse Behind: Nurses Working with disAbilities

iUniverse books may be ordered through booksellers or by contacting:

iUniverse
2021 Pine Lake Road, Suite 100
Lincoln, NE 68512
www.iuniverse.com
1-800-Authors (1-800-288-4677)

ISBN-13: 978-0-595-39649-8 (pbk)
ISBN-13: 978-0-595-84053-3 (ebk)
ISBN-10: 0-595-39649-6 (pbk)
ISBN-10: 0-595-84053-1 (ebk)

Printed in the United States of America

To my daughter, Lauren.
My life and the world are so much richer because of you.
I love you BIG.

The person who says it cannot be done should not interrupt
the person who is doing it.

—*Chinese Proverb*

Contents

Welcome to Florida:
A Parable for Nurses Who Become Disabled

By Donna Carol Maheady, ARNP, EdD

At some point in time, most parents of children with disabilities come across the "Welcome to Holland" message written by Emily Perl Kingsley in 1987. The message originally appeared in the Los Angeles Times, *in Abigail Van Buren's "Dear Abbey" column. For those who aren't familiar with the story, it's about someone who plans a vacation to Italy but ends up in Holland instead. This story has guided my life as a parent of a child who is disabled and my work as a nurse and nursing educator. Below, I have adapted this message for nurses who become disabled.*

I am often asked to describe the experiences of nurses who become disabled—to try to help people who have not shared that unique experience understand it and imagine how it would feel. It's like this...

Imagine planning a fabulous trip to New York City after graduating from nursing school. You plan to work at a prestigious medical or research center there. You buy a new stethoscope, lab coat, scrubs and medication handbook. You plan to work as a staff nurse and eventually get promoted to unit manager of a busy intensive care unit or emergency department. On your days off, you are eager to visit the Statue of Liberty, Ellis Island and the Metropolitan Museum of Art. You can't wait to see the bright lights, Time Square and Broadway. It's all very exciting. After months of eager anticipation, the day finally arrives. You pack your bags, and off you go. Several hours later, the plane lands. The flight attendant comes in and says, "Welcome to Florida."

"Florida?" you exclaim. "What do you mean Florida? I signed up for New York! I'm supposed to be in New York. All my life I've dreamed of going to New York. I'm not old enough to move to Florida!"

But there's been a change in the flight plan. The plane has landed in Florida, and there you must stay. The reason is that you have a disability.

The important thing is that they haven't taken you to a horrible, disgusting, filthy place, full of pestilence, famine and disease. It's just a different place.

So you must go out and buy new guide books. And you need to learn a whole new language—the Americans with Disabilities Act, vocational rehabilitation, reasonable accommodations—and perhaps go back to school for an advanced degree. You may need to buy some new equipment and learn new ways of performing your nursing skills. But a bonus will be that you will meet a whole new group of people whom you would never have met.

Florida is just a different place. It's slower-paced and less flashy than New York. But after you've been there for a while and you catch your breath, you look around and begin to notice that Florida has beaches, warm weather, magnificent sunsets and palm trees. Florida has the Salvador Dali and Morikami museums. And it has patients who *still* need your care—in hospitals, nursing homes, health departments, schools, community centers, camps, case management, infection control, administration, teaching and research positions.

But everyone you know is busy coming and going from New York City. And they're all bragging about what a wonderful time they are having as nurses in New York. For the rest of your life, you will say, "Yes, that's where I was supposed to go. That's what I had planned."

The pain of that will never, ever, ever, ever go away, because the loss of that dream is very significant.

But if you spend your life mourning the fact that you didn't get to New York City, you may never be free to enjoy the special, lovely things about being a nurse in Florida.

Acknowledgement

Blessings and thanks to all of the nurses who had the courage to share their stories. It has been an honor and a privilege to come to know all of you. Special thanks to my husband, Tom Gili, the architect whose love and support serves as a foundation for my life and all of my work. And to Cynthia Gomez and Lisa Foulke, for their patience and editorial skill in helping me knit together the pieces of this book, my thanks as well.

May the wind always be at your back.

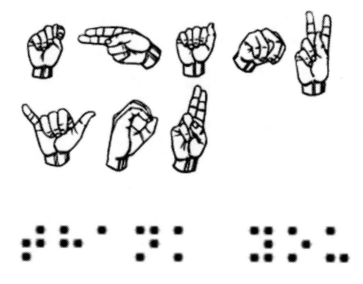

Preface

By Donna Cardillo, RN, MA

I love to read biographies of famous and successful people, especially those I admire. These books remind me that everyone, no matter who it is, has had obstacles to overcome in his or her life. True stories of courage and triumph over adversity, of beating the odds and proving the naysayers wrong, keep me buoyant and centered in my own life. Such stories serve to nudge me forward as I strive to develop myself personally and professionally, always looking for bigger and better ways to fulfill my mission on this planet, face my fear and self-doubt, and move forward in spite of them. Although the nurses who are featured in this book are not famous, their success stories are as powerful as any I've ever read or heard.

Leave No Nurse Behind: Nurses Working with disAbilities is groundbreaking work. I applaud Donna Maheady and all of the contributors for their courage and honesty in bringing these stories to light—for telling the truth about their struggles with disabilities and related prejudices, celebrating their indomitable spirit and determination, and doing things many others have said they could not do. However, the book is not just about nurses with disabilities. There are messages here for all nurses—in fact, all people. The central message is that anything is possible when you set your mind to it.

I once read a quote that said, "If someone tells you that you can't do something, it's probably because they're afraid that you will do it." If I listened every time someone cast doubts on my plans, aspirations, or abilities, I'd be nowhere, doing nothing. One of the biggest life lessons I've learned is that where there is a will, there is always a way. Simply put, if you want something badly enough, you'll find a way to make it happen no matter what the circumstances. A strong enough desire or sense of passion for something, along with a firm belief in oneself and one's work, can move mountains, part waters, change minds and laws, and make things happen.

Many of us develop tunnel vision and only see one way to do something. If that way becomes blocked, we have a tendency to become frozen in place. Yet, there is always another way, another door to go through, another approach, and another path to follow. As evidenced in this book, the sheer will and determination of the human spirit, not to mention the resourcefulness of nurses, is astounding. A nurse with a mind made up is a powerful force to reckon with. I've seen it and experienced it time and time again. Rather than thinking, "I can't do this," these nurses think, "How can I do this?" proving that persistence and determination will always win out in the end.

Nurses are versatile and multitalented. We possess a great body of specialized knowledge, experience, and skills even right out of nursing school. Likewise, nursing is a broad and multidimensional profession. Fortunately, there have never been more opportunities for nurses to use that specialized knowledge and skill to make a difference—whether at the bedside or in nontraditional nursing positions. If one work setting or specialty isn't right, there are plenty of others to choose from. There is something for everyone, no matter what his or her needs, in this glorious profession.

This book is a true testament to the creative and resilient spirit of all individuals, but especially nurses. As you read each incredible story, you will marvel at not only the strength and character of each nurse, but also at the innovative way he or she managed to overcome hurdles. Sometimes the obstacles placed by society are greater than those created by nature.

Read this book, and then read it again. Share it and recommend it. Use it as a resource for information and advice. Keep it handy for reference when you need inspiration, energy, motivation, and a nudge to move forward in your own life. Tell the stories to others. We are nurses—a proud, strong, and substantial group. Let's celebrate and support all nurses and the profession of nursing as a whole.

Donna Cardillo, RN, MA
President, Cardillo & Associates
Creator of Career Alternatives for Nurses™

Introduction

By Donna Carol Maheady, ARNP, EdD

Often, I think of nursing as a gift—something that I use in the care of those in need. It is more than a profession or a job. I was born to be a nurse. It's who I am, not what I do. I experience nursing as a vocation or calling—a privilege. Perhaps it is in my heritage. Because of my parents' divorce early during my childhood, I lost touch with my large, Irish family. Recently, we reconnected, and I learned that many of my cousins became nurses. Whatever the reason, I am so proud to say, "I am a nurse."

Much of my past has influenced the course my life has taken. I grew up in the 1950s in a low-income housing project in Hartford, Connecticut. I saved my babysitting money to buy the uniform needed to be a Candy Striper at Mount Sinai Hospital. I lived, played and went to school with children of all faiths and colors. My mother, sister Karen and I attended the local Congregational Church. I have an old photograph of me in a snowsuit with my mother on a church retreat led by our interim minister, a young seminarian named Andrew Young. He later went on to become a noted civil rights activist who worked with Dr. Martin Luther King, Jr. Often, I think that the seeds of my activism for the disabled were planted during that retreat.

I now have a daughter, Lauren, who is mentally disabled and has been diagnosed with obsessive-compulsive disorder, autism and epilepsy. My advocacy efforts grew from Lauren's needs and spread over time to benefit many other people with disabilities. I serve on numerous disability-related advocacy boards and committees. For me, helping nurses with disabilities has evolved into a unique practice area, one that focuses on caring for our own. I have learned that where you stand is indeed where you sit.

This book grew from my experience writing *Nursing Students with Disabilities Change the Course* along with my work creating and maintaining the nonprofit website www.ExceptionalNurse.com. I have taught nursing since 1982; and over the years, I have met many students with disabilities. I'm a pediatric nurse practitioner with a particular interest in disabling conditions. My doctoral dissertation studied the experiences of nursing students with disabilities, and I have written articles related to nurses and nursing students with disabilities.

Through the stories of so many nurses I have come to know, I have learned that I am not alone in the way I feel about nursing. These stories demonstrate continuous self-sacrifice, devotion, a missionary spirit, and love and tenderness for others in spite of personal pain or suffering. These nurses practice nursing in spite of the odds.

The current nursing shortage has brought many issues about the nursing profession to media attention. One group of nurses and potential nursing students continues to be left out—nurses and students with disabilities. Countless numbers want to study to become nurses or continue to practice as nurses. Many face enormous challenges in order to be granted the opportunity to do the work they love. Exact numbers of nurses with disabilities are not available for many reasons. Some nurses do not disclose their disability due to fear of termination. Others are involved in lawsuits and have been advised not to share information.

For varied reasons, employers and academic programs have turned nurses and nursing students away. "Essential functions" and "lifting and CPR requirements" are strictly enforced by some employers and programs. Employers often state safety and liability concerns as a basis for not hiring or accommodating a nurse with a disability. However, Sowers & Smith (2002) reported there exists no data to suggest that health professionals with disabilities pose any greater safety risk to their patients.

The National Nurses Survey (2000) reported that 9,438 nurses listed disability or illness as a reason for having an occupation other than nursing. Anecdotal reports show that nurses have disabilities that mirror the general population. Additionally, nurses have been injured by lifting patients, through violence inflicted by patients or exposure to latex, hepatitis and HIV.

Nurses are intelligent, caring and creative problem solvers. Daily, they assist patients in navigating the healthcare system and adjusting to disability and other health concerns. Common sense informs us that nurses with disabilities have much to offer patient care. They can identify with a patient's thoughts, feelings and concerns.

In most practice settings, nurses help each other and work as a team. They barter and seek the expertise of colleagues when needed. "Can you check my IV while I'm in room 204?" "Can you catheterize Mrs. Smith? I'll help you change the dressing on Mr. Coleman." "Can you help me turn Mrs. Garcia?" In addition, nurses accommodate colleagues who are pregnant by changing assignments so as not to expose them to communicable diseases or by hanging blood for nurses who can't do so due to religious beliefs.

Why does it become such a challenge to accommodate nurses with disabilities in the same way? Reasons are numerous. Regulations became more stringent over time. Core performance standards and specific physical attributes became part of admission to nursing programs, and "essential functions" became part of nursing job descriptions. In an effort to improve patient safety and uphold high admission and retention standards, the profession became more selective.

The Americans with Disabilities Act was passed in 1990 in an effort to level the playing field for people with disabilities. The law and the meaning of reasonable accommodations have been interpreted differently over the years, resulting in inconsistencies in admission and hiring decisions. Nursing students with disabilities have been admitted to nursing programs and graduated. In other cases, students with disabilities are denied admission. Anecdotal reports show that nurses with disabilities are being hired and retained, and some are receiving remarkable accommodations. Many other nurses with disabilities are pushed or nudged out the door. Policies and attitudes vary greatly from one institution to another.

This book presents the stories of nurses with a wide range of disabilities who have continued to work. The book focuses on the *abilities* of these nurses, not their limitations. It does not provide a solution to all of the issues related to disability within the nursing profession. However, it does provide the opportunity for 11 nurses, who happen to have disabilities, to share their stories of success and triumph. Their stories show how nurses can turn a disability into an integral part of their nursing care—a force of giving in spite of the odds stacked against them.

The stories in this book demonstrate how nurses with disabilities do their work with and without accommodations, often by reinventing themselves. If they can't get in the front door, they go around to the side door. Often accommodations can be simple and low in cost. Sometimes all a nurse needs is for a colleague to extend a helping hand.

Working helps nurses with disabilities maintain independence, health and self-esteem while benefiting patients. Some work with service dogs, and others use wheelchairs and special equipment. Often, they work in flextime positions. But at the end of the day, they have worked—for patients and for themselves. After reading the book, the reader will be sure to ask: "Where can I find a nurse like one of these to care for my loved ones and me?"

This book is important for nurses at any point in their careers. Reading these stories should give nurses greater insight into the experience of nursing colleagues who become disabled or those who are hired with a disability. It is also vital reading for administrators and nurse managers working with nurses applying for positions or requesting accommodations.

Employing nurses with disabilities is a win-win situation. Nurses benefit, patients benefit and the nursing shortage may be, to some extent, reduced.

State boards of nursing should consider these stories as they work to address issues related to nurses with disabilities. The stories also provide information for nursing educators, nurses, administrators and vocational rehabilitation counselors. They answer the often-asked question: "Will a nurse or student with a disability be able to find a job?"

This book will help nurses with disabilities become more resilient and encourage continued practice. It will inspire more students with disabilities to consider nursing as a career. And it will help employers and nurse managers become more open in considering reasonable accommodation requests from nurses.

Finally, nurses need to consider the possibility of illness or disability in their career planning and recognize that staying as healthy as possible, being flexible, continuing to obtain certifications and advanced degrees, and maintaining a positive attitude will increase their employability options. Disability doesn't always mean the end. Often it is the beginning. If it happens to you, don't be defined by the disability; be defined by how you handle it. Now, let's get to work.

◆   ◆   ◆

Maheady, D. (2003). *Nursing students with disabilities change the course*. River Edge, NJ: Exceptional Parent Press.

Sowers, J., & Smith, M. (2002). Disability as difference. *Journal of nursing education, 41* (8), 331-332.

U.S. Department of Health and Human Services, Bureau of Health Professions. Registered nurse population from the 2000 national sample survey [WWW page].
URL http://bhpr.hrsa.gov/healthworkforce/reports/rnsurvey

1

Reasonable Accommodation: Legal Protection for Nurses with Disabilities

By Susan B. Matt, RN, MN, JD

A Legal Introduction

Until just over a quarter of a century ago, individuals with disabilities were considered incapable of contributing to the economy. There were no legal protections for these people in the workplace, and a nurse with a disability was rarely—if ever—heard of. With the passage of the Rehabilitation Act of 1973, the climate began to change, and the Americans with Disabilities Act of 1990 gave nurses and other workers with disabilities a weapon to fight the discriminatory practices that prevented them from obtaining and keeping employment.

The purpose of this chapter is to raise awareness about the rights of nurses with disabilities in the workplace and to provide some commonly accepted accommodations as examples to emulate.

The Rehab Act prohibits discrimination against individuals with any handicap by any entity receiving federal funding. Section 501 applies to the federal government, Section 503 to companies that do business with the federal government, and Section 504 to recipients of federal financial assistance. Thus, any healthcare employer receiving Medicare payments or that is in any way connected to the federal government or federal funding is covered under this law.

Enacted to further level the playing field for people with disabilities, the ADA incorporated most of the standards established under the Rehab Act. Title I of the ADA protects individuals with disabilities in the workplace.

Despite numerous attempts to narrow the protections available under these laws, the core legislative intent remains intact. Under both acts, employers are required to provide reasonable accommodation to qualified individuals with disabilities. Under the ADA, however, as in other federal antidiscrimination laws, an employer is not covered unless its workforce includes "15 or more employees for each working day for each of 20 or more calendar weeks in the current or preceding calendar year" (42 U.S.C. § 12111(5); Clackamas v. Wells, 2003). But even those employers not covered under the ADA are still required to meet this standard under the Rehab Act.

Qualified Individuals with Disabilities

The Rehab Act and Title I of the ADA were enacted to protect "qualified individuals with disabilities" in the workplace (42 U.S.C. § 12101 *et seq.*; 45 Code of Federal Regulations, 2002; U.S. Equal Employment Opportunity Commission, 1992). But what constitutes a qualified individual?

According to the ADA definition, a qualified individual with a disability "meets the skill, experience, education and other job-related requirements of a position held or desired, and who, *with or without reasonable accommodation*, can perform the essential functions of a job" (42 U.S.C. § 12111(8)).

The law specifically defines "disability" with respect to an individual as:

(A) having a physical or mental impairment that substantially limits one or more of the major life activities of such individual;

(B) having a record of such an impairment; or

(C) being regarded as having such an impairment. (42 U.S.C. § 12102(2)).

Since 1992, when the Equal Employment Opportunity Commission published its ADA Technical Assistance Manual, the U.S. Supreme Court has considered a number of cases involving disabled employees. Its rulings have altered the definition of the term "disability," limiting the population protected by the ADA (Sutton v. United Airlines, Inc., 1999; Murphy v. United Parcel Service, Inc., 1999). As a result of these decisions, the manual's addendum advises that "[w]hether a person has an ADA 'disability' is determined by taking into account the positive and negative effects of mitigating measures used by the individual" (EEOC, October 2002).

In practical terms, this means that if one has little or no difficulty performing any major life activity as a result of use of a "mitigating measure," such as hearing aids or medication to control a disabling medical condition, one may not meet the ADA's first definition of an individual with a disability.

The courts rely on the Rehab Act regulations issued by the Department of Health, Education and Welfare in 1977, which define "physical impairment" and "major life activity." Physical impairment is considered "any physiological disorder or condition, cosmetic disfigurement, or anatomical loss affecting one or more of the following body systems: neurological; musculoskeletal; special sense organs; respiratory, including speech organs; cardiovascular; reproductive, digestive, genito-urinary; hemic and lymphatic; skin; and endocrine." (45 CFR § 84.3(j)(2)(i) (2001)). The HEW Rehab Act regulations provide examples of major life activities that include walking, seeing, hearing and performing manual tasks. (45 CFR § 84.3(j)(2)(ii) (2001)).

Bottom line? For individuals to be protected by the Rehab Act and the ADA, they must have a physical or mental impairment that substantially limits one or more major life activity *and* must meet the job qualifications and be able to perform the essential functions of the job *with or without reasonable accommodation.*

Reasonable Accommodation

Assuming that a nurse meets the initial criteria of the ADA, the key consideration for employment is "reasonable accommodation." For an employer to be required to provide any accommodation, the nurse must first ask for it. An employee cannot remain silent and expect the employer to bear the initial burden of identifying the need for and suggesting an appropriate accommodation (Matt, S.B., 2003). The ADA states under Title I that "reasonable accommodation" may include—

(A) making existing facilities used by employees readily accessible to and usable by individuals with disabilities; and

(B) job restructuring, part-time or modified work schedules, reassignment to a vacant position, acquisition or modification of equipment or devices, appropriate adjustment or modifications of examinations, training materials or policies, the provision of qualified readers or interpreters, and other similar accommodations for individuals with disabilities. (42 U.S.C. § 12111(9))

The reasonableness of an accommodation depends upon a common sense balancing of the costs and benefits to both employer and employee (Lyons v. Legal Aid Society, 1995).

An accommodation may not be considered unreasonable merely because it requires the employer to assume more than a minimal cost or because it will cost more to obtain the same overall performance from a disabled employee. An employer is not required to provide accommodation if it presents an "undue hardship." This is defined as requiring significant difficulty or expense when taking into consideration a number of factors specific to the covered employer's business (42, U.S.C. § 12111(10)).

How does one go about deciding where the line is separating reasonable accommodation from undue hardship?

If a specific situation requires reassignment to accommodate the disability, the employer is required to comply. However, the employer is not obligated to reassign the nurse to a better position than he would normally be entitled to, nor is the employer obligated to provide the accommodation the nurse requests or prefers if an alternative reasonable accommodation is offered (Henricks-Robinson v. Excel, 1997; Schmidt v. Methodist Hospital, 1996).

Furthermore, seniority takes priority over disability in reassignment requests. So if a nurse is reassigned to a "light duty" position because he cannot lift patients, another nurse with seniority may request such reassignment, "bumping" the nurse with a disability (US Airways v. Barnett, 2002).

Under the ADA, reasonable accommodation is required in three aspects of employment:

1. to ensure equal opportunity in the application process,

2. to enable a qualified individual with a disability to perform the essential functions of a job, and

3. to enable a disabled employee to enjoy equal benefits and privileges of employment (EEOC, May 2002).

Examples of some acceptable accommodations in each category relevant to nurses follow.

The Application Process

The application process can be quite challenging for a nurse with a disability. Without reasonable accommodation, an opportunity may be lost due to misunderstandings. To prevent such a scenario, a nurse with a moderate hearing loss may require an assistive communication device. Let's say the applicant requests provision of a Pocket-Talker, a device that amplifies sound during one-on-one interactions. This meets the ADA requirement of reasonable accommodation by mitigating the effects of the applicant's hearing disability and allowing him or her to effectively communicate during the interview process.

It is important to be aware that there may be reasons directly related to a disabling condition for an employer to deny employment. One that could apply to the healthcare field has already been addressed by the courts, which have maintained that the ADA permits an employer to refuse to hire an individual because his performance on the job would endanger his or her own health due to a disability (Chevron U.S.A. v. Echazabal, 2002).

Consider as an example a nurse with an immune deficiency condition who is denied employment in a facility that provides health care to individuals diagnosed with a variety of infections that, if contracted by the nurse, would endanger the nurse's health. In such a scenario, an employer may be legally permitted to deny employment.

Performance of Essential Functions

An employer is not obligated to decrease performance standards as an accommodation, nor is it required to provide personal use items, such as hearing aids (EEOC, May 2002).

Provision of auxiliary devices and services is included in the ADA mandate. Examples of such devices and services for nurses who are deaf, hard of hearing or who have other communication-related disabilities include, but are not limited to: telecommunication devices for deaf individuals (TDDs, also referred to as TTYs) for communicating by telephone; sign language and oral interpreters (not necessarily practical in a nursing environment, but may be acceptable in an educational or other work setting); computer-assisted real-time transcription (CART) services (also may be impractical in a nursing setting); note takers for training courses and meetings; captioned training tapes; and assistive listening systems.

In a situation where a nurse cannot hear blood pressure sounds, a digital blood pressure device may be sufficient accommodation. Technological advancement has provided medical professionals with a variety of tools to accommodate hearing disabilities, including stethoscopes that function to translate sounds into visual displays, permitting nurses who are hard of hearing to "hear" heart and lung sounds.

It may be necessary to redefine the job duties as a reasonable accommodation. An employee must be able to perform the essential functions of the job, but where it is possible to remove certain nonessential tasks from an employee's work requirements, it should be done.

In some nursing units, shift reports are provided using a tape recorder. These recordings are often impossible for a nurse with a hearing loss to hear and understand. As reasonable accommodation, the employer might require a face-to-face report that would allow the disabled nurse to use speech-reading skills to supplement his or her hearing.

Nurses are often expected to lift and turn patients in acute care and long-term care settings. For a nurse with physical limitations that preclude him or her from performing such tasks, it may be possible for the employer to reassign those tasks to another worker, such as a nurse's aide. This may be more readily accomplished in a larger facility with more extensive staffing than in a smaller one with minimal staff. As detailed earlier, any accommodation is not "reasonable" if it results in "undue hardship" for the employer.

Some nurses work in settings other than direct patient care. For nurses working in an office setting (i.e., telephone triage), physical changes to the workplace might be necessary. For example, a desk might be lowered to accommodate a wheelchair, or the employer might provide a nurse who is hard of hearing with an amplified telephone.

Nurses with certain disabling medical conditions may require breaks at specific times to monitor blood sugar levels, self-administer medications, or avoid extreme fatigue. An employer should ensure that regularly scheduled breaks are provided as accommodation and make allowances for needed relief on an emergency basis.

Equal Benefits and Privileges of Employment

It may be necessary for an employer to make physical changes to the workplace to enable an employee with a disability to enjoy the benefit of an employee cafeteria or break room. Such changes may include installing a ramp or lowering the sink to enable a mobility-impaired person to enter the area and reach the sink. If the employer provides a television in the employee break room, the employer would be required to provide an infrared assistive listening device or captioning to enable a hard-of-hearing employee to enjoy the same benefit of hearing the television enjoyed by other employees.

Summary

Wading through the legal requirements of disability laws is no easy feat for the nurses requesting accommodations or for the employers that must decide whether such requests are reasonable. As is the case with most legal issues, the laws that have been enacted to protect the rights of individuals with disabilities are fraught with standards that are difficult to interpret. Furthermore, there are cases in the courts brought by those who would have these laws taken off the books.

The legislature intended to eliminate discrimination against people with disabilities in all areas of life. Nurses with disabilities are entitled to request and receive reasonable accommodation to enable them to perform the essential functions of a job. Furthermore, they have the right to equal enjoyment of the benefits and privileges of employment enjoyed by others. By knowing the law, nurses with disabilities can ensure that they are afforded the same opportunities available to other nurses, thereby benefiting the general population needing the care of a competent, compassionate nurse.

Susan B. Matt, RN, MN, JD, is an attorney whose practice encompasses disability law as well as guardianships and family law issues. Susan earned her juris doctor from the University of Washington in Seattle. She earned her BSN from the College of New Rochelle in New York and a master's in neuroscience nursing from the University of Washington. Her career took her from the bedside to administration and risk management, which ultimately led to her interest in law. A passion for disability law grew from her severe hearing loss. Susan is a student in the University of Washington's doctoral nursing program, where her research focus is on nurses with disabilities. She lives with her husband of 32 years, the last of her four children and a menagerie of pets. She can be reached at suzimatt@u.washington.edu.

◆   ◆   ◆

42 U.S.C. §12101 *et seq.*

45 Code of Federal Regulations §84.3 (2001, 2002).

Chevron U.S.A. Inc., Petitioner v. Mario Echazabal, 536 U.S. 73, 122 S.Ct. 2045, 2002.

Clackamas Gastroenterology Associates, P.D., Petitioner v. Deborah Wells, 123 S.Ct. 1673, 2003.

Henricks-Robinson v. Excel, Case No. 94-3156 (D.C.D. Ill. 1997).

Lyons v. Legal Aid Society, 68 F.3d 1512 (2nd Cir. 1995).

Matt, S.B. (2003). Reasonable accommodation: What does the law really require? [WWW page]. URL http://www.amphl.org/articles/matt2003.pdf

Murphy v. United Parcel Service, Inc., 527 U.S. 516 (1999).

Schmidt v. Methodist Hospital, 89 F.3d 342 (7th Cir. 1996).

Sutton v. United Airlines, Inc., 527 U.S. 471 (1999).

The U.S. Equal Employment Opportunity Commission. (2002). Federal laws prohibiting job discrimination questions and answers [WWW page]. URL www.eeoc.gov/facts/qanda.html

US Airways, Inc., Petitioner v. Robert Barnett, 535 U.S. 391, 122 S.Ct. 1516, 2002.

U.S. Equal Employment Opportunity Commission (January 1992). *A Technical Assistance Manual on the Employment Provisions (Title I) of the Americans with Disabilities Act.*

U.S. Equal Employment Opportunity Commission (October 2002). *A Technical Assistance Manual on the Employment Provisions (Title I) of the Americans with Disabilities Act Addendum.*

2

Get Over It! Nursing with Multiple Sclerosis

By Sheila Sirl, RN

I've talked to many nurses who say they always knew they wanted to be nurses—that they never considered being anything else. For me, nursing was one of about a million different things that I wanted to do. I didn't even enter nursing school until I was in my 30s. But I can look back to my childhood and see the women who, for me, defined what a nurse is. Three of my favorite aunts were nurses—all different, but all alike at the same time. They had a concern for others, a sense of humor and "two feet on the ground" style common sense. Once I started nursing school, I knew I had found the vocation that would define me, no matter what I did to earn a living.

I was raising three children—all teenagers—when I was going through school. My husband was great. He remained patient as I put in 10 to 12 hours of class and study each day. One room of our house was even designated the "study room."

My study group would spend hours huddled inside, calling out for pizza and often working far into the night. I loved it all: the learning, the doing and sharing it with others who wanted to be nurses as much as I did.

When we needed to spread out our books, we spilled out into the dining room and sunroom. My family withstood it all. And when it was done, my husband and daughter were on the auditorium stage to present me with my pin at the capping ceremony. My two sons were in the balcony doing a two man "wave."

No matter how frustrating my job became on any given day, I never questioned my decision to become a nurse. I worked in hospitals, home care and long-term care. I loved each setting. My specialty became working with people affected by Alzheimer's disease and other forms of dementia. Eventually, I moved into nursing management, but I stayed in settings where I could continue to have plenty of patient contact.

I truly loved what I did. It became not just what I did, but who I was. I believed that my career would only end when I was ready to end it.

The career that I had worked so hard for and so loved began to unravel with a bout of sudden muscular weakness. I had previously overlooked some symptoms that I now know were significant. But the weakness couldn't be overlooked.

I called my internist when the weakness was discernable but still benign. I was driving into work and could barely make it. My hands would periodically drop off the wheel and onto my lap—though fortunately never both at the same time. I called her as soon as I got into my office. I was scared. She insisted that I get someone to drive me in immediately and warned that I should be prepared to go into the hospital. That only scared me more. I had hoped to hear her chuckle and tell me to relax.

I spent three days in the hospital. They had no idea what was wrong with me. Although I never regained my full strength, I began to feel a bit stronger. The neurologist gave me the old standby answer: "Maybe it's stress."

I just wanted to go home and go into denial, so I agreed. In all fairness, mine was a stressful job. So I handed in my resignation. I left a job I loved more than any I'd ever had. I thought that if I went back to working as a staff nurse, without management responsibilities, I would be back to normal in no time.

I went through two more jobs in the next year, all the while getting worse. Finally and reluctantly, I left nursing altogether. By that point, I needed a cane to walk without falling, was fatigued all the time and still had no idea what was wrong.

Even without the stress of work, the symptoms continued to pile up. When I began experiencing Lhermitte's sign (tingling down my back when I tipped my head forward), the doctor sent me to another neurologist. He performed what was perhaps the worse neurological exam I've ever had—and I've had plenty—then asked me how my marriage was. Needless to say, I was furious.

I hadn't asked for this. I hadn't even asked to see him. By the time I got home, though still angry, I used my visit with him to go into full-scale denial.

Things were a bit easier when I wasn't working. I even mustered the energy to open a bookstore and coffee shop on the village square with my husband. It was a fun venture; and with our daughter-in-law acting as manager, I could spend much of my time just enjoying the customers and doing what work I could.

But eventually the symptoms returned. When they did, I broke down and went to an internist. I warned her that if she sent me to another idiot I'd just go home and wait to die, and it would be on her head. I could always muster a traditional melodramatic Irish threat when it was needed.

The neurologist she sent me to this time told me that I had multiple sclerosis. There was no beating around the bush. He sent me for tests to confirm it, but he was confident in his diagnosis.

I had primary progressive MS. In less than a year, I was in a motorized wheelchair. I was approved for Social Security disability on my first application. As much as I needed the money, I hated that it carried with it the title "disabled."

As difficult as it was to admit I was really disabled, I was so weak and fatigued those first couple of years that I could barely take care of myself. We had to close the bookstore. I couldn't imagine going back to work, let alone wonder if there would be a place for me to return to should I ever choose to try.

Still, I didn't let my nursing license lapse. I used courses by mail to keep up with my continuing education, and I faithfully renewed a license I didn't know I'd ever need again. I couldn't hang on to my driver's license quite as easily, and for the first time since I was 16, I didn't have the freedom to just pick up and go.

It has been said that the disability minority is one of the few that anyone can suddenly join. No matter how healthy people are or how many miles they jog each day, everyone is just one drunk driver or one MRI away from becoming part of the disabled minority. I was now a part of that community, like it or not.

I don't think my self-image ever suffered from the physical changes, but the loss of a career I loved—especially when I had no idea if I would ever be able to work again—did a real number on my ego.

I went through the usual MS routine. I tried the injectable medications with little success, had periodic rounds of IV steroids, and went through a million different treatments for symptoms until the right combination was found. My whole life seemed to revolve around my health. I adapted to losses, then readapted when things changed again. Sometimes I slipped so quickly that I wondered each night what the following morning would be like. "Would I wake up and be unable to move out of my bed?" I thought. I didn't see an end to the losses. Without my faith in God and the support of a spectacular family, I don't know how I would have coped.

Then something happened. I realized one day that I hadn't really lost any ground in more than six months. Some of my fear was slipping away. Maybe I wouldn't end up in a nursing home after all. I also started to feel more energy. I actually felt that I could be productive again and began to look beyond the concerns of my body to a bigger world. When my health remained stable for almost a year, I decided it was time to do something. I realized that I might stay the same for the next 20 years. I didn't want to look back and see that I had wasted two decades simply waiting to get worse.

I called the Social Security Administration and told them I wanted to retrain and go back to work. Looking back, I find it interesting that at that time, I never even considered the possibility of using adaptations to continue working as a nurse. Now, several years later, I am fighting against that very attitude in the healthcare industry.

I was sent to the Bureau of Vocational Rehabilitation to develop an educational plan. After an initial informational meeting, I was assigned a case manager, a lovely lady named Nina, who proved to be very encouraging and supportive. The community college from which I had received my nursing degree had recently sent out letters to the nursing graduates encouraging them to come back for a legal nurse consultant certificate program. I had always been interested in law, so that was the path I chose.

Nina was somewhat doubtful after reading my medical reports. She wondered if I could do it. I found myself in the unexpected position of having to convince someone that I could come off disability payments and go back to work. No one knows what will happen tomorrow, and there was no way I could guarantee that I would remain healthy enough to complete my schooling and go back to work. But then who can, with or without MS? All I could guarantee was that I wanted to succeed, and I would work as hard as I could to do so. Even as I worked to persuade her, I heard a voice in the back of my mind saying, "Gee, I hope I'm right."

I convinced her and was enrolled by the next semester. I arranged to use the county dial-up bus service to get to and from school. It dawned on me the first day I went to classes that it had been two years since I had gone anywhere without a family member. My daughter called that evening to see if I was okay. I felt like I was starting kindergarten all over again—only now my daughter was hovering over me like a mother hen.

I quickly fell into a routine. Nothing is as easy when you're doing it from a wheelchair, but I took figuring out ways to do things differently as a challenge. To this day, the creative problem solving that goes with adapting to life on wheels is something I enjoy.

The more I did, the more I felt ready to try. I've always been a reasonably confident and outgoing person, and as I got past the initial strangeness of functioning from a wheelchair, my confidence began to return. I've even found many advantages to my situation. I love kids; and now that I'm on their level, I find they love dealing with an adult who always looks at them eye-to-eye. I never have to worry about ironing the back of my shirt or jacket. I frequently get to sit at the head of the table in business settings because it's usually the easiest choice. And I must admit, I love the feeling of power.

I know some of that may sound silly, but it reflects an attitude change that was essential for my survival. I knew I had to look at reality and deal with it. I couldn't change my circumstances, but I knew I could keep from letting them change me for the worse. People ask how I can remain positive. My answer is always, "Would grousing and complaining change my circumstances?" Of course not. Then I'd just be a cranky, defeated person in a wheelchair. I'd be a victim of MS. Instead I choose to be a woman who happens to have MS and who refuses to be a victim of anyone or anything.

One of my biggest attitude changes needed to be in the area of adaptive equipment. I've often heard people say, "I'll do anything not to be in a wheelchair." I've even thought it myself. This can be a productive attitude when there is something you can do to keep yourself walking, such as after a stroke or accident. However, when the condition that makes a wheelchair necessary can't be changed, it can be a self-defeating attitude.

At the time when I was again moving out into the world, I probably could have lived without a wheelchair. However, I would have been limited to moving from my bedroom to the family room and into the bathroom when it was necessary. There are prisoners in maximum security who get more freedom than that. I never could have gone to school or work under those circumstances. Now I can look at my adaptive equipment as no more or less than the tools I need to remain active and independent; it's no different from the glasses I've been wearing since I was 8 years old.

I had to find the right combination of supportive equipment and the routine that would allow me to maximize my available energy. I learned that the procrastination, which comes so naturally to me, had to be avoided at all costs. When you can't be sure how much energy you will have tomorrow, you have to do as much as you reasonably can today. I always had papers and research done early. I never knew if I would have a bad day or two and wanted to be prepared for that. Actually, my energy level remained pretty good throughout my schooling. Pacing myself kept me from crashing.

When I was almost ready to go back to work, it dawned on me that I could probably drive with hand controls. It was time to replace our lift van anyway. I mentioned this to my doctor, who immediately referred me to a driving clinic. There, a great guy named Terry conducted an evaluation and determined that there was no reason why I couldn't do it. He trained me to drive again. At first, it felt odd to use my hand to accelerate and brake, but it didn't take long at all for it to become as natural as driving the old way had been.

I worked with the Bureau of Vocational Rehabilitation to have the state pay to have my van adapted. A few years earlier, my husband had returned to work in the telecommunications industry so we could preserve our retirement account. But he was laid off shortly after the September 11th attacks. This left us in tight financial circumstances. We were living on my humble Social Security checks, those retirement funds we couldn't avoid tapping and credit cards. Paying for the van would have been a stretch.

My rehabilitation counselor was great, and I got my van in time for my job hunt. I do admit though, that my being a "nudge" didn't hurt. A hands-on approach is key to getting the system moving for you. I would frequently call and find out where things stood. If they were at a standstill, I'd find out where the problem was, and then I'd call someone to push the process along.

I can't stress enough the importance of taking control of your destiny in this respect. When you have to adapt your life to a major change brought on by a disability, you have to deal with hoards of people, agencies and providers, and most of them are completely overwhelmed. It isn't that the people you deal with don't care. The majority of them do. But like so many of us, they are doing the job of two or three people. Let those people know you appreciate their efforts, but also be assertive enough to make sure things are getting done.

So there I was, ready to begin a career as a legal nurse consultant, once again an independent driver. My husband said I was acting like a 16-year-old with her license for the first time. I would run any errand just to get behind the wheel and go.

For the first time in many years, I had the experience of sending out my resume. After so many years of an overabundance of unfilled nursing positions, I forgot how it felt to have to actually go out and look for work.

My rehabilitation case manager gave me the names of two vocational placement specialists to choose from. I went on gut instinct and chose Pat, who turned out to be a wonderful help. She coached me on interviewing. We focused especially on those aspects of the process that related to my disability. If you have an invisible disability, you have no obligation to reveal it, as long as you can do the job you're applying for. But when you come rolling in on wheels, you can't very well keep it hidden.

Pat and I touched on all of the things that could have potentially put off a prospective employer. Even though you are protected by the ADA, it can be hard to prove someone didn't hire you because of your disability.

Each person has to find what works best in his situation. I found what worked best for me was addressing any concerns the employer had up front. When I was setting up an interview, I would let the individual know I was in a wheelchair. This way I could find out about the accessibility of the building as well as give the person a few days to get used to the idea. I didn't want the person who would be interviewing me to be so distracted by the surprise that he couldn't concentrate on getting to know me. It also gave the interviewer time to formulate questions relating to my circumstances so that I could answer them during the interview, rather than having questions come up after I left.

As trite as it may sound, when you believe you can do something, others tend to believe you can as well. For that reason, much of my preparation for finding a job was convincing myself that I could do whatever I needed to. In reality, there is very little I can't do. I just have to find new ways of doing it.

Because my resume contained both my nursing education and experience and my legal nurse consultant education, I received calls related to both. Even though I was excited about everything I'd learned about law, I didn't rule out any leads. But almost universally, when recruiters from the medical field heard that I was in a wheelchair, their interest in me quickly cooled. I felt badly about this. Most of the jobs were in management and were easily within my capabilities. I believe this may reflect the tendency for those in the healthcare field to see anyone who is physically challenged as "sick" and in need of care, not someone who can give care.

I finally got a call from an attorney who was not the least deterred by my wheelchair. He needed a legal nurse consultant, and he needed one quickly. Because he was interested in having someone who would work as an independent contractor, the distance between my home and his office didn't put me off. I would be able to work at home some days, taking in other work as it came along. I accepted his offer, and I haven't regretted it yet. I have a great deal of contact with clients, which gives me the opportunity to interact with people—an aspect of nursing that I had loved. And since much of my work with them involves solving problems or advocating, my need to help others is met.

Traveling around downtown Cleveland, where my job often takes me, is an interesting challenge. I have a file case on wheels. I strap my laptop case on top of that with a bungee cord, and then I push the whole thing ahead of me to get from the parking garage to the office. I lovingly call this device my "crap on wheels." Needless to say, people notice me. They also give me a clear path. But I've never been shy, and I rather like challenging their image of how a person can deal with life.

I keep my RN license up-to-date, and if the time and the opportunity were right, I would certainly welcome the chance to get back into a traditional bedside nursing position. I also feel strongly about the need for the healthcare industry to find a place for disabled nurses.

All the disabled nurses I've met say they've learned a lot about how to care for people from what they've gone through. These nurses are a valuable resource, and healthcare is poorer for their loss. So often, the barriers keeping these nurses out of jobs are arbitrary. Job descriptions imply "essential functions" that the employee would never be called upon to do. The result is that people who could do the job are excluded for no good reason.

The ADA states that a person cannot be denied consideration for a job provided that he can do the essential functions of the position. It also states the employer is responsible for providing reasonable accommodation for the person to be able to do the job.

The description for the post of director of nursing in a large hospital may include such things as the ability to perform CPR or to provide bedside care. Because these things sound as if they are noble expectations, they often go unchallenged. But in reality, you would be hard pressed to think of a situation in which those things would actually be a part of the nursing director's day in a large facility.

It can be hurtful to hear the lament of the healthcare industry that it can't find enough nurses, when you are there, ready to work, but found "not good enough anymore." With a little creative thinking, many nursing positions could be filled. The necessary accommodations are often much simpler than employers think. Perhaps flexible scheduling in situations where direct patient care is not involved would fill that management position. Since most healthcare settings are—or certainly should be—physically accessible for anyone with a special need, workspace adaptation may involve little more than rearranging furniture.

There is even a place in direct patient care for many disabled nurses. In settings that are more residential than clinical, is there really a reason why a nurse can't work from a wheelchair? Perhaps it would be a problem if there were not other medical personnel on the floor to handle what emergencies might occur. But often an individual in a chair can do anything they are called upon to do, if they are allowed to try.

When I look back on the jobs I did as a nurse, I can honestly say that with some simple accommodations, I would still be able to do most of them. I could still assess patients, pass medication, do patient teaching and prepare care plans, all from my wheelchair. Many settings use care teams. A creative assignment of duties within a team could provide a much-needed registered nurse to a facility, as well as a much-needed job for a disabled nurse.

All nurses, whether they have a limiting condition or not, are individuals, with their own strengths and weaknesses. The individuals who do the hiring need to look at potential employees that way, without making assumptions based upon the label of "disabled." If an individual has physical or mental limitations, ask how they will handle the aspects of the job that are of concern.

A disabled nurse looking for work also has a responsibility to examine the job she is seeking. She should look at what is involved and then realistically assess her ability to do the work. It's important for the nurse to go in with a good idea of any accommodations that may be needed, as well as a good idea of how she may deal with any special challenges. Perhaps the most important thing a disabled nurse can do for herself is to form her own self-image. Don't allow others to define you, and don't assume you can no longer do something until you've explored all the possible ways you may be able to accomplish it. Finding a new way to do an old task and discovering some way to overcome a limitation can be a wonderfully creative challenge.

I had a bumper sticker on my wheelchair for a while that read, "Get Over It." It's a phrase I was famous for while raising my kids. Following my diagnosis, it became a phrase I needed to keep saying to myself. It is so easy to fall into the trap of self-pity and to spend countless hours reviewing what you've lost, instead of thanking God for what you have. Sometimes you have to just kick yourself in your mental behind and *get over it*. It's not that it makes you more pleasant to be around, or that it makes others more comfortable, or any other selfless reason. Do it because you will never be able to get on with your life if you don't.

I've come a long way from that fearful place I was in when everything seemed to be unraveling around me. My faith, my family and some wonderful support people have made a huge difference in my life. I can now honestly say that my MS is no longer the looming monster it initially was. When I'm tempted to worry about what will happen tomorrow, I remind myself that even before I had MS, I didn't know what would happen tomorrow.

Sheila Sirl, RN, was born and raised in Cleveland, Ohio. She attended a Catholic grade school and a Catholic girls' high school. Sheila has been married for 35 years. She and her husband have three children and seven grandchildren. Sheila went back to college and got her nursing degree when her children were teenagers. She has worked in hospitals, home care, long-term care and parish nursing. Sheila lives with her husband in a semi-rural community about 40 miles east of Cleveland. She can be reached at ssirl@adelphia.com.

Work*able* Wisdom

- **Live life to the fullest.** You can spend your life measuring how much you've lost or lost out on, or waiting—as with conditions like MS—for a disability to worsen. Or you can value all you have remaining and work creatively to make the most of your abilities.

- **Self-advocate.** Sheila demonstrates the importance of "nudging" things forward to get the necessary services.

- **Meet employer concerns head on.** By addressing any concerns they may have about your ability to perform essential job functions and reassuring them about your abilities, you don't leave them wondering after the interview is over.

- **Be open to learning new skills.** Whether it is learning to be a legal nurse consultant or driving a car with hand controls, a positive attitude will help a nurse with a disability return to work or continue to work.

3

Hill, What Hill? Nursing with Guillain-Barré, Osteoarthritis and Lifelong Obesity

By Lynne Shaw, RN, BSN, MBA, CNA, c-MSEM

For those of you who have a tendency to come down with a "case of the vapors," you had better sit down now and take out a cool cloth and fan! This fact may come as a shock to many people, especially those of us in the healthcare profession. But seeing that I call the shots as I see them and don't sugarcoat the facts, I'll say it: *Nobody is perfect.*

Okay, are you breathing again and over needing a dose of Atropine? Yep, it is the truth. And isn't it a wonderful thing that we aren't perfect? Imagine how boring life would be if we were all perfect—void of our flaws, differences, uniqueness, quirkiness and individuality.

What would we do when we couldn't complain? Everyone has something they cannot do well. Actually, we each have many things we don't do well, but we don't admit many of them, even to ourselves. Yes, I am afraid that we must face the fact that everyone goes through life with a handicap, whether or not you play golf. Some of us have several handicaps. The difference lies in deciding if you are going to let your handicap help you win in the grand game of life or blame it for losing.

Now the second shock (Crank up the defibrillators!): Life ain't fair! *Gasp!*

I do hope you figured this one out before you left your teenage years. Some of us have had a few more struggles and hills to climb than others. Or at the very least, the hills were just a little more obvious than the hills of those around us.

I've been climbing my first hill since the day I was born. It is the Hill of Fat. Yes, it took me a long time before I was able to say that word, instead of using less offensive words like chubby, plump, full-figured, heavyset, big-boned—and the more vivacious definition—voluptuous! Of course, I was all of those things. Growing up a fat kid, it wasn't until I was in my youthful 40s that I became a BBW—Big Beautiful Woman.

But just as soon as I had become comfortable with my now more socially acceptable body size, my body decided to play painful tricks on me and remind me that while my mind was still a youthful 40-something, the rest of me was not getting any younger and would soon be needing replacement parts.

Let me tell you a little bit about myself. I am now a glorious age 50, and I have been a nurse for almost 29 years. While in college earning my nursing degree, I became an EMT. I had a great time jumping in and out of ambulances and falling in love with the stars of TV's "Squad 51."

My career has afforded me some wonderful opportunities. I worked as a nurse's aide through high school and college, and when I became a registered nurse, I wound up working as a trauma/ER nurse. I loved it. When I was young, most of the jobs for girls were as nurse's aides, cashiers or waitresses. I was always the one in Girl Scouts who came to everyone's assistance. In a crisis, I was the only one who didn't scream or faint.

I think I got "the calling" somewhere between Junior and Senior Girl Scouts at a two-week overnight summer camp. The urge to help people came naturally to me. Visions of white uniforms and those perky little caps began dancing in my head. (I admit, the cap lasted all of four hours my first night on duty in the emergency department!)

I have also had the privilege of being an emergency department manager and house-wide nursing supervisor in a large medical teaching center in Boston. It's a post I continue to hold today. Along the way, I put in 20 years as an EMT and taught EMT courses. I worked as a police dispatcher for 12 years part-time, and I was one of the first female firefighters (Yes, boots, coat, helmet, hoses, fire trucks—the works!) way back in the 1970s. I proudly served my community for 15 years. Along the way, I served on a disaster medical assistance team, worked in five hospitals in three states, plus did a winter stint in Florida as a "snow bird," before going back to school to earn my master's in business administration.

I currently hold an adjunct professor position at the same college teaching disaster management studies to master's-level students, and I am a student myself, earning a second master's degree in emergency management. I plan to pursue a doctorate in emergency management before the end of the decade. I think I am one of the few people at the college who is a faculty member, alumna and student all at the same time. In addition, I am active in my town and own a disaster management consulting firm.

Now, on to the personal side of my life. I grew up as an Army brat, so I've traveled extensively over the years. I have a small but very close family consisting of my sister, her husband and my two nephews. I share a log home with three house cats, two house bunnies, and down the road, the large member of the family—a Chincoteague Pony. So you can see, I do not live a sedentary life.

Why do I share all of this with you? Because these aspects of my life and the love of my family are the reasons that I never gave up when the hills grew into mountains.

Another hill to climb appeared in the form of a disease called Guillain-Barré. I ended up in my own emergency department and intensive care unit when I was 25. There's nothing like being on the inside of the bedrails and completely dependent on others for every bodily function to make you realize what you put your patients through.

Luckily, I climbed that hill. Now at the other side, I have minimal deficits to show for my ordeal. While it's not a journey that I would have chosen and not one I ever want to relive, it was a learning experience. I know it made me a better nurse.

The hospital I worked for at the time was instrumental in helping me remain productive. As days of recovery grew into weeks and months, the hospital assisted by allowing me to do some work from home. We were readying for our first Joint Commission on Accreditation of Healthcare Organizations visit as a new facility, and I wrote the emergency department policy and procedure manual. When I was able to return to work, they allowed me to work four-hour shifts, then six hours, and then eight hours three days a week until I could do the full 40 hours.

This facility was also very accommodating to other staff members with disabilities. It was the first time I ever worked with a nurse who was "imperfect." She had a malformed hand. Looking back, I remember several clerical employees who used wheelchairs, a hospital runner with a paralyzed arm who had a carry tote, and several others with canes or leg braces. No one seemed to take much notice, and everyone did his job.

It wasn't until my early 40s that my body decided again to scream "mutiny." Having inherited my mother's osteoarthritis, my knees began to make a lot of noise and cause me a great deal of pain. I recall my mother barely being able to walk some days during her early 50s. This was before the anti-inflammatory drugs, routine joint replacements, arthroscopies and the like. Momma died at the age of 59 from a massive heart attack while being treated for liver cancer. She was the kind of woman who, on a good day, you could not keep up with. On her bad days, she rested quietly and rarely uttered a complaint.

I learned to be self-sufficient early in life as I took over many of the household duties and became a partial caretaker for her when she was not feeling well. From my dad, I learned organization and delegation. This was a man who could pack a family of 10 in a Volkswagen Beetle and still have room for the luggage and dog. From my mother, I learned how to regroup and rethink quickly when things did not go as planned. And I learned to smile through the pain and continue marching.

By this time, it was clear that my many years of nursing, crawling around in burning buildings, jumping on and off of ambulances, fire trucks, and the occasional rescue boat and helicopter had damaged my knees beyond repair. I had found that I could be an ED nurse manager without putting too much strain on my knees and body, so I worked in that capacity for six years. When I later became an administrative coordinator for nursing, I found myself in a job that required—and still requires—covering 27 floors in five buildings for a total of about 2.5 miles of walking during any given shift.

In 1997, the pain and discomfort of the osteoarthritis in my left knee required an arthroscopy. That bought me relief for about 18 months. By early 1999, the pain in the right knee was so severe that I needed to use a cane almost all the time, including at work. I am not one to take anything more than acetaminophen or ibuprofen. But those were not controlling my pain, even when I took more than I should have. Most days, I was in tears at some point. However, I did not miss any work. In fact, I continued to teach college one night a week and run my consulting business.

Within the year, I'd had two arthroscopies on the right knee. I was back to using the cane. It was time to take some drastic steps. Making rounds in a certain number of hours and responding to codes, emergencies and fire alarms had become next to impossible. After a discussion with my orthopedic surgeon, he wrote a letter to the hospital. It stated that I had to either leave my current position or be given a scooter as an ADA accommodation. I also got a handicapped plate for my vehicle.

I considered my job options. I could be a case manger or a nurse reviewer, or I could take some other desk job, but at the time those were hard to find. And they didn't interest me.

I approached the hospital with my accommodation request. I can't say that they immediately wrapped up a scooter for me and happily gave me the key. But after some discussions, they finally purchased a scooter for me for use at the hospital.

I did have to research the scooter market, choose the scooter myself and present a written rationale and financial justification. I carefully explained the cost of losing an experienced supervisor, which included advertising and coverage costs, as well as the cost of orienting a new employee.

The approval process took several months. In the meantime, my right knee continued to deteriorate. In June of 2000, I had a total knee replacement. The scooter arrived while I was on sick leave. Initially, I was to be out of work for 15 weeks. When I told my surgeon that the scooter had arrived at the hospital, he allowed me to go back to work after seven weeks. I was overjoyed at being able to get back to work. I had to use crutches for another few weeks. My peers had let the staff know that I would be returning on a scooter. To my surprise, it made little difference to anyone.

It took some creative thinking to find places to park and a place to "garage" for recharging the scooter when I was off duty. After some trial and error, those issues were solved. After a few weeks, I went back to my cane. I decided to make it part of the wardrobe, so I found a multicolored, hand-crafted wooden one at a craft fair and promptly named him "Fred." Since he and I were going to be buddies for a long time, I decided to declare him a friend rather than a foe.

It was somewhat of a novelty for the patients, and each group of new interns and residents gave me an initial second look. I also became the go-to person for advice for staff, patients, families or physicians seeking information and advice on getting a scooter.

I struggled internally with my need for the scooter. Partly, the struggle was due to the realization that I was not as young as I used to be, and I couldn't do everything I once had. At times I felt that I was being punished for something. I think that's a normal response for anyone who has suddenly found herself in a situation like this. I had certainly felt that way when I was diagnosed with Guillain-Barré.

But I had the support of my family and friends. My sister reminded me of how much pain and suffering my mother must have endured quietly. I felt that I had to show our mother that her daughter didn't succumb to the pain any more than she did. The support of my coworkers and staff was wonderful.

My disability didn't decrease the amount of work I did. Rather, I seemed to have been put on a few more committees. When on duty, I still did short walks around the floors and units once I got to the area. Even while on the scooter, I still was able to (and I loved to) help the staff as much as I could with patient turns and pull-ups, handing equipment, starting IVs, etc. I was just careful to make sure my interactions would not hinder the patient or the patient care.

Despite my limited physical capabilities, I still think like an ED nurse and manager and still respond in emergencies as I've always done. When I looked at the patients we cared for, I realized how lucky I was to be there doing the job that I loved. I had no reason to give in or give up.

In 2002, the Hill of Fat started reminding me that it was still there. A few other health issues related to my weight also began to surface. During that year, I had built a new home and moved to the same town in which my family lived. I'd had a successful consulting year and had continued teaching and working on my second master's degree. I was commuting one hour and 40 minutes to work four times a week.

Now I was struggling again with knee pain, hip pain and back pain. I had blood pressure issues, sleep apnea and a few other maladies. I seriously thought I was going to die before the end of the year. But on Christmas Eve, I found a way to climb the hill once and for all. I made one of the major decisions of my life. In June of 2003, I underwent a laparoscopic gastric bypass.

Where am I now? As of 2006, I have maintained a loss of 90 pounds. I no longer use the scooter, although it is parked ready for anyone else who may need it. I am off all my medications, except those that post gastric bypass patients must take for life. I have almost no joint or bone discomfort at all. I walk everywhere. I can walk two to three miles a day, climb stairs, clean my horse stalls, lift 50-pound bags of grain, work in my yard, and even shovel snow. I would still like to lose another 40, but I feel happy, healthy, lucky and fortunate to have been given the opportunity to make this change in my life.

Growing up in a career military family, Lynne Shaw, RN, BSN, MBA, CNA, c-MSEM, was born in Virginia and moved to Munich, Germany, before settling in Massachusetts. She received her nursing degree from Fitchburg State College, a master's in business administration from Anna Maria College and is currently completing a second master's degree in disaster emergency management at AMC, where she is also an adjunct professor. Lynne runs a consulting business offering disaster management services to the healthcare industry. She has been a registered nurse for 29 years and is also a retired firefighter. She has worked in community hospitals, trauma centers and teaching hospitals. She currently works as a nursing supervisor in a teaching hospital in Boston. Lynne lives 80 miles from the hospital, in the country, with her six pets. She can be reached at Quabhcc@aol.com.

Work*able* Wisdom

- **Be realistic about what you can and cannot do professionally.** Being a nurse requires above all that we never compromise a patient. That doesn't change just because you do.

- **Accept it for what it is, then move on.** Grieve if you need to. Get angry, cry and get it out of your system. Then look at how you are going to deal with it. After all, nurses are creatures of creativity and problem solving.

- **Prepare if you can.** If you know you will be dealing with a disability in the future, prepare now by looking at what your options may be if you remain in nursing. If you will need assistive devices, start learning about them now and how they work. Talk to people who are similar to you or have been where you will be. Learn from their experiences.

- **Present your case for accommodations professionally.** If you need to request accommodations, think beforehand about how you will present your situation professionally and factually. Be aware that use of assistive devices, depending on your job title and function, may also be governed under OSHA. Be ready to present the rationale of the mutual benefits to you and the company assisting you in meeting your job requirements through accommodation.

- **Do the best with what you have.** If you must give up your clinical role due to lack of mobility or another barrier, then think of using your skills to teach others. You can write or be an entrepreneur, a legal nurse consultant or any type of nurse consultant. You can also do case management—the possibilities are boundless.

4

Am I Handicapped?
Nursing with One Hand

By Susan Elaine Fleming, RN, BSN, MN, CNS

Many people feel that they were destined for a career in nursing. I am one of those people. My destiny was to be a nurse. Growing up in the 1960s in a Los Angeles suburb and sandwiched between two brothers, playing outside meant playing "Army." I gave my rifle—a birthday present—to my brothers so that I could play "the nurse." Our backyard became a neighborhood fort. As my older brother was entering kindergarten, I watched how he learned to tie his shoes. At 4 years old, without giving it much thought, I taught myself to tie my shoes with one hand.

My mother, grandmother, aunts and uncles were teachers. So they were at a loss in advising me about nursing. But they shared with me the story of my great grandmother, who was a nurse. At the turn of the century, my great grandmother found herself divorced and the mother of two children—a newborn and a 2-year-old. It was then that she developed her nursing skills.

Living in the boomtown of Seattle, Washington, she recognized a hospital shortage and wanted to help. She put two hospital beds in her living room and soon was delivering babies and recovering the mothers in her own home. She was well respected by the local medical community. She was able to financially care for herself and her children. At a very young age, I chose to follow this road for my future vocation.

The reality that I was different did not come to light until I entered kindergarten. I came home after the first day of school and said to my mother, "I was the only one in my class missing a hand. Why didn't you tell me?" She replied, "You didn't ask."

I knew from that day forward that I would experience the world differently than others, and that I would have to adjust.

On Saturday mornings, I would watch cartoons. I remember one morning seeing a commercial depicting 10 sad-looking children with various handicaps. There it was—a young girl just like me—missing a hand! The announcer urged viewers to help the handicapped through monetary donations. Later that day I asked my mother, "Am I handicapped?"

She looked at me and said, "Only if you want to be." Those words set me free. I knew it was my choice and that I was not destined to a life of sadness and begging.

The sterility of the '50s and '60s was evidenced by a world of segregation. People who were different in color, mental status or who were physically challenged were often placed in schools and institutions away from the public. Children without disabilities were sheltered from the dim realities of the world. I remember children actually getting nauseated if they saw my hand. During school dances, when other children held hands on the dance floor, I knew my place was next to the teacher. However discouraging these experiences, I gained strength.

Then adolescence arrived. I felt that I was the only one in the big wide world that was different. I refused to wear my artificial hand. I felt that people needed to accept me the way I was. Mind you, I always offered to carry everyone's coats and sweaters to cover my missing hand. I was fortunate to have dear friends with whom I could share my feelings. However, I really did not discuss my hand.

In tenth grade, I was finally able to take German, a language skill that I had been working on since first grade. The first week, I sat in class with my hand under the desk bundled in a sweater. That's when my greatest nightmare happened. The teacher, unaware of my missing hand, asked, "What happened to your hand? Did a shark bite it off?" That was it! I left the classroom and did not return.

At the age of 15, I left high school and went to an alternative school in the morning, working as a nurse's aid in the afternoon. I worked in a home for the severely retarded and disabled. At $1.35 an hour, I felt "in the money." I soon went to work for an agency. One night I was sent to work at an acute care hospital. I loved it. I knew that two character traits of mine were courage and compassion. And I liked physical work.

I ended up working as a nurse's aid at a local community hospital. The nurses and doctors were always encouraging me to go to school and become a registered nurse. The idea appealed to me.

At 17, I graduated high school early, and I was ready for college. I enrolled in a community college and dropped by the nursing department. I was told that I would not be eligible for their program. I continued with college and at age 19 received an associate's degree.

In addition to working as a nurse's aid, I took on some jobs in accounting. I was totally discouraged. I hated the solitude and the lack of physical movement of office work. I knew that I wanted to help people and work with others. I went back to college and took anatomy, physiology and microbiology.

Even though I wanted dearly to be a nurse, I knew others might block my path. I approached the same nursing school again. This time they agreed to test me to see if I could perform the kinds of tasks required from a competent nurse. The nurses at my local hospital generously gave me their extra supplies so that I could practice at home. Still, I failed the test and was told that I "would endanger a patient's life."

I felt that I would be a nurse's aid the rest of my life. That was a better option for me than working in an office. I was content. Yet, I knew that I shouldn't let someone who only knew me five minutes make a judgment that would affect the rest of my life.

One day one of the older doctors asked how my goal of becoming a nurse was going. "Not well," I replied. I told him my story. He advised me to go to the Los Angeles County Hospital School of Nursing.

There I found a group of culturally diverse faculty members. Could it be that these women and men had faced their own challenges in the workplace and in college? I believe this is true. I asked if I needed a "skills test." They told me that it would be illegal. They could not create a test that could specifically eliminate me from the program. Today, this constitutes "singling out" and is illegal. I thought about my past experience and was disheartened.

I was admitted that spring and began classes in the fall. I thought about other people with disabilities who might attend my previous school. I didn't want their dreams shot down.

I called the Office of Civil Rights in San Francisco. They sent a woman to talk to the president of the school. She interviewed the president, the nursing school faculty and me. She told me that she could tell that the school personnel were lying, but she could not prove it. The nursing school had told her that they had given me extra support to help me get through nursing school. This, of course, was untrue.

This was completely twisted. But with no proof, I dropped the complaint and decided to move forward and direct my energy to completing my nursing program at Los Angeles County School of Nursing.

I hit nursing school with great ambition. I was voted class president during my first month. Soon, I landed a job in the local emergency department as a student nurse worker.

At first I was a little nervous that I might not be able to do all the tasks asked of me. But everything turned out great. Still, I waited for the Big One—the one skill that would stop my progression to graduation. My pediatric instructor saw my uneasiness. She told me that my fear of not being accepted would not stop here. After graduation, there would be the job interviews to maneuver and new positions to master.

Being a nurse allowed me the opportunity to live where I wanted to. Within six months after graduation, I headed to the Pacific Northwest. It was there that I met my future husband. He later joined the Army, and we spent the next 10 years moving from Washington State to Texas to Hawaii and on to Germany. I worked every place as a nurse and still managed to give birth to four children. These frequent moves allowed me to challenge myself in very different ways.

Even with my left hand completely missing, I became competent in starting IVs, giving injections, performing CPR and applying sterile dressings. As an accommodation, I use a hemostat and keep scissors in my pocket, along with a large pair of sterile gloves. But I also found that all nurses—with or without dis- abilities—had their own weaknesses and strengths. We all needed each other. I learned to humble myself and ask for help when I catheterized patients. In return, I always tried to offer my help when it was needed. I think nurses would have been resentful if I had been a drain to the team. This is even more true today with the increase in patient loads.

My experiences with patients have been priceless. On one occasion, I was working on a medical floor of a large Army medical center. I was asked to accom- pany a fragile patient to the x-ray department. As I sat in the waiting area with the patient, I saw a technician run out of an examining room screaming "He's coding!" At that moment I made an uncomfortable decision to leave my patient and entered the room. I found a large man frothing and "bull dogging" on the table. I immediately started CPR, grabbed a mask and assisted the patient with ventilations. As people moved into the room, I delegated tasks, started an IV and helped transfer the patient to the ICU. I found out later from the tech that the patient I had left in the waiting room had done just fine.

That evening as I went home, I thought about the fears voiced by the nursing school that had turned me down, that "I would endanger a patient's life." I had in fact saved a patient's life. From that day forward I purged those hurtful words from my consciousness.

I currently work on a mother-baby unit. Most of my time is spent assessing, planning and implementing care of mothers and babies. I am sometimes with a patient or couple who has just heard the tragic news that their baby has been born imperfect. I listen attentively to the couple's comprehension of what has taken place and for their readiness to hear my story.

On one occasion, my patient and her husband had just learned that their son was born with an unusually small, fragile body. They expressed how they were drawn closer to Jesus. I told them that we all have crosses to bear. Some of us are born with a built-in cross. I explained how my own cross became a blessing. When I was young and dating, some young men could not accept my hand. However, my husband was different. After 20 years, he has shown love and acceptance of my many imperfections. My missing hand acted as a "meter" of sorts, keeping me single long enough to meet the right man.

Because of our military life, I got to work at many hospitals. That gave me the chance to reflect on the reactions from other nurses to my "blessing." I must say that almost all of the nurses that I have worked with have been great. When I initially start on a new ward, the nurses are usually a bit apprehensive. Then I show them my bag of tricks, which includes tying my shoes with one hand and starting IVs. Soon enough, they begin to focus on my abilities as a team member and quality nursing care.

There is a wealth of opportunity in the healthcare industry as society welcomes more and more workers with disabilities. If we show kindness and compassion to one another, our patients benefit. In turn, patients will view the healthcare system as a kind and more compassionate organization.

Susan Fleming, RN, BSN, MN, CNS, has been practicing as a registered nurse in hospital settings for more than 20 years. She received her BSN from Washington State University's Intercollegiate College of Nursing, Spokane, and her MN and CNS from the University of Washington. She is a clinical nursing instructor at WSU's Intercollegiate College of Nursing. Her clinical specialty is maternal/child nursing. She won the 2005 Cherokee Uniforms Inspired Comfort Award. Susan is married and lives with her four children in Chewelah, Washington. She is a board member of www. ExceptionalNurse.com. Susan can be reached at sefleming@wsu.com.

Work*able* Wisdom

- **Exercise patience and an open mind.** An open mind is essential to recognize that skills can be preformed safely and effectively in many different ways. Patience is necessary to understand that a nursing student or new nurse may need time and practice to develop certain skills.

- **Do not let someone who doesn't know you dictate your future.** If you are a student or nurse with a disability, don't let yourself be discouraged by disparaging words from someone who has known you for five minutes.

- **View yourself as a valuable team member—not a drain.** No apologies are needed. Everyone has his own weaknesses and strengths. Yours may just happen to be more visible.

5

A Late Bloomer: Nursing with Rheumatoid Arthritis and Bipolar Disorder

By Cary Jo Cook, RN, CMSRN

My path to nursing was long and circuitous. I graduated from nursing school as a registered nurse when I was 36 years old. Previously, I had worked as a credit manager for about 10 years. Then, after a hiatus from working, I took a part-time job as an emergency veterinary assistant and as a full-time wildlife rehabilitator. A friend from the vet clinic, where I worked for four years, was planning to attend nursing school, and she encouraged me to do the same. Her name was Carey. I looked at all her materials from school. I knew that I had a strong interest in helping people who suffered from mental illness. Before I knew it, I was in nursing school and loving it. My mom had suggested nursing to me when I was in high school, but back then I'd had no idea what nursing really was.

Since becoming a nurse, I have worked in skilled care, behavioral health, med-surg, neuroscience and ICU step-down. I've also served as an agency nurse. I currently work in an orthopedic spine surgeon's clinic as a nurse clinician.

I experienced my first joint problems in junior high school: bursitis in a heel and bilateral knee chondromalacia with patellofemoral syndrome, both of which continued into high school and limited my participation in gym class. I even had to have a bunion shaved off my right foot when I worked as a waitress at the age of 15. As a young adult, the knee pain continued. I had swelling and generalized joint pain and intermittent redness.

Finally it got bad enough that I had to start seeing doctors. At times, I was symptom free. But at other times I could be a 25-year-old healthy, fit woman who could barely walk up a step due to severe knee pain. I saw a few internists and orthopedists over a period of around 10 years. None could give me a diagnosis or help with the pain. A year or so after I became an RN, I had a severe episode; the swelling was so bad that I could not open medication bottles or insert an IV. I was certain I had rheumatoid arthritis. I referred myself to our hospital's most popular rheumatologist.

This rheumatologist diagnosed me with RA as well, and soon I started a regimen of multiple medications. They helped a little but not enough. But within a short period of time, I began taking Remicade infusions.

This was the beginning of the end of my hospital career. I improved dramatically on the Remicade and did pretty well for about a year. I struggled with fatigue constantly, so I eventually had to cut down to one full-time job—up until that point I had been working beyond full-time while raising a teenaged boy as a single parent.

I transferred to a newly opened neuroscience unit at a sister hospital and had critical care classes and training along with extensive neuroscience training. This last year in hospital nursing, I moved up from staff nurse to clinician. I worked as a day charge and worked on the step-down unit. I loved neuroscience nursing, and I didn't want to leave it.

However, a combination of upper management difficulties at the hospital and my ever-worsening RA made it clear that I could not continue spending 12 hours or more on my feet every shift and lifting patients who were often twice my size. The fatigue and the hand, wrist and foot pain and swelling were just too much. I never wanted to be known as one of those nurses who just sits in the station and doesn't take care of her patients, let alone help others with theirs. I decided to leave the hospital and find a job that was less physically challenging.

I took what seemed like a great job at a 13-surgeon orthopedic practice. I became the spine surgeon's nurse, which seemed to dovetail nicely with my neuroscience knowledge, experience and enthusiasm. But I didn't realize that in a surgical private practice, it is all about the surgeons. Add a PA to the mix, and there isn't a lot of need for nursing assessments, at least not currently where I am.

There are also general orthopedic patients with fractures and strains. This has required that I learn how to cast. The problem here is the cast saw. I did not anticipate the cast saw. It's a heavy, awkward, vibrating device used to remove casts. It causes me great pain in the hands and wrists. I am very lucky that the doctor and PA with whom I work are very kind about doing cast removal for me when I ask. Neither of them acts like they are annoyed or resentful. I am grateful, because like most nurses, I don't like to ask for help. RA causes chronic tendonitis as well as the obvious joint deformities, so often I just don't have the strength or control to work this machine. I think the patients would be alarmed if I appeared to have a difficult time handling the saw on their extremities.

Presently, I feel underemployed. Mentally, I am not challenged. I do not assess patients; the PA and surgeon do that. Occasionally, I get to give some advice over the phone or refill some prescriptions. Once in a while, I can triage by telephone a bit. It is really frustrating to have all of this nursing knowledge and not use it. Unfortunately, in the hospital setting, knowledge is not enough. The hospital nurse must also be the physical equivalent of a construction laborer. Therefore, my knowledge, enthusiasm and experience are not being used in the setting where they could do the most good.

My second disability is not disabling at this time, but it needs to be discussed for the benefit of others. I am bipolar. This is a huge and frightening admission for a person in healthcare to make, even or especially to other healthcare workers. My symptoms began in high school. At that time, I was living in a dysfunctional family setting and was what many would call a wild child. I stayed out late, smoked pot, drank excessively and was generally self-destructive. It was—and still is—hard to separate the mood swings from everything else and find a starting point for this illness. But I suspect it appeared when I was 15.

I was not from the type of family who would hospitalize or institutionalize a teen for bad behavior, so I was not diagnosed. As a 21-year-old, I was diagnosed with post-traumatic stress disorder. I kept having flashbacks. I was using drugs, living with friends and without a car, but I still somehow managed to hold down a menial job.

I met a nice Air Force boy and married him. I stopped drinking and using drugs, detoxing at home. This was when I started having hints that my so-called wildness might not be my biggest problem. In retrospect, I had quite obviously been self-medicating.

We soon had a son and were thrilled. But I would have mood swings or bouts of depression that I just didn't understand. Life went on. When our son was 3, my husband and I separated. The mood swings started to spiral out of control. My son and I stayed with my parents while I worked full-time during the day and went to a business college at night. I wanted to provide a better life for my son and me.

My now-ex-husband and I worked hard to remain on friendly terms. We came up with our own joint-custody arrangement, so our son saw each of us every week, pretty much on whatever schedule our son wanted or needed.

Sleeping and eating became erratic, sort of all or nothing. I took care of my son, but I didn't take care of myself. When my son was with his dad, I went on the occasional date. Sometimes I acted wildly. Even I could see I was getting out of control.

Following a bad breakup with a boyfriend, my mood swings intensified. I was working as a credit manager for a newspaper chain. Sometimes I would be sitting at my desk completely overtaken by a desire to physically bash my head against the wall. These compulsions became very strong. I also wanted to crash my car into something like a brick wall or maybe drive off a highway overpass.

I kept all of this to myself because, of course, it sounds crazy. I thought I could hear some sort of whispering, far away and quiet. I could not discern what was being said, but I would sort of cock my head if no one was looking and listen really hard to try to make it out. I was terrified. I thought I had schizophrenia. Then I knew little about the disorder, but I knew schizophrenics heard voices. I made an appointment with a mental health practitioner.

I was diagnosed with bipolar disorder. Within about five minutes of my first therapy appointment, although the visit was much longer, I was prescribed a boatload of medications. I wasn't told about any side effects. I took a week's leave of absence from work and left my son in the care of my ex and my parents. I went to my sister's house to stay, take the meds and try to get my head straight so that I could return to work. But the medications turned me into a zombie. I could not eat. I went from a size eight to a size four within a matter of weeks. I was tired. And I couldn't think straight. My doctor changed the meds.

I had started dating a guy from work and soon we moved in together. He took care of me while my doctor tried to find the right combination of medications for me. I was on Lithium for quite a while, along with antidepressants. I began gaining weight but the lethargy made it difficult to work and think. I quit and took a year or so off from work. Finally I decided to give up the Lithium. I was very careful to eat and sleep, and my family watched me for "nuttiness." I was taking only an antidepressant, and I was doing well.

I took the job at the vet clinic. I had a couple of hypomanias. They were treated short-term with Risperdal or Depakote, but never for more than about a week. I just couldn't tolerate the stuff.

After a couple more years, I started nursing school, and I graduated with high honors. I got straight As in all my nursing classes.

I continue to take antidepressants, and I probably will for life. I sink into a big depression every time I try to stop. I haven't had a mania since before starting nursing school, and I have now been a nurse for more than five years. I couldn't be more stable on medications; it may even be that the bipolar disorder burned itself out, as sometimes happens as people age.

When we got to our behavioral health unit in nursing school, it was our final semester. I got along well with my classmates and my instructors. I heard a lot of disrespectful misconceptions, mainly due to fear of the unknown from the other students, as we prepared for clinicals on the psych unit.

I talked to my instructor, Jackie, and decided to "come out" to my fellow students about my bipolar diagnosis. Until now, I had kept it a deep, dark secret. My fellow students were stunned when I got up in front of the class and gave a first-hand account of the disorder. I was afraid that people would treat me differently or even attempt to prevent me from getting licensed. But I felt it was more important for my fellow students to understand that people with mental illnesses are human beings just like them.

I tried to explain that individuals with mental illnesses like mine were just unfortunate enough to have a chronic condition that affects the brain instead of the body. I think my ploy worked. My friends were much more compassionate at clinicals than they had been when initially discussing mental illness in class.

I have never asked for or received any formal accommodations. I was raised in such a way that it is terribly embarrassing to have RA or bipolar disorder. We just don't get sick, and when we do, we suck it up and get back to work. It has been one hell of an adjustment for me to even admit to myself I have a chronic illness.

What I have received is help on a personal level. On the medical-surgical unit, my coworkers would help me spike a bag on a bad day or open a tough blister pack of meds. When my hands and wrists were weak, my coworkers did the majority of my lifting for me. I also asked my floor director not to assign me any patients with tuberculosis, since exposure to TB is contraindicated while on certain RA meds like Remicade. This wasn't a problem, as we didn't get many patients with TB anyway. Of course, when anyone else needed help, I was always the first to volunteer, whether it was a difficult patient, passing meds or taking over so someone could have a crying jag in the restroom. That is what team members do for each other, and I was very lucky to work with the kind of people who helped each other out.

Very few people know about my bipolar disorder—even now. It isn't a problem for me anymore. But before, every mistake or misstep I made would have ever after been met with the whispered comment, "Well, she is bipolar, you know." I have seen similar situations and did not want to go there myself. I told a very select few people and never a supervisor. I feel it is good to have someone who knows. I would certainly want to be alerted to not being on top of my game if someone thought that was the case. (See Appendix B, Disclosing Your Psychiatric Disability to an Employer.)

Patient safety should always come first. I would quit nursing before I would work in the midst of a mania and do something that could hurt or kill someone. There is no excuse for irresponsibility when other lives are at stake.

At my current job, I also receive personal accommodations, as I mentioned earlier. My surgeon and physician's assistant are very nice about the cast saw—my biggest issue. I did not tell them I had RA when I started working at the clinic. I honestly didn't think it would affect my work. I am able to use the cast saw at times—it just depends on whether I'm in the middle of a flare or not. We lug around a heavy laptop computer as well. When my hands are in pain, the PA and surgeon carry it for me. They are terrific and never complain. I'm sure they have no idea how much those little helping hand moments mean to me. No one wants to feel disabled.

Nurses with disabilities understand better than anyone what it is like to be ill or injured—and what mountains of worry a patient is often buried beneath. These are the nurses who relate better to the patients on a personal level because of their shared experiences. These are the nurses who better understand the big picture—the ramifications illness or injury may have on a patient's entire life. It cannot be emphasized enough what a comfort these nurses are to their patients.

Cary Jo Cook, RN, CMSRN, grew up in Clinton, Iowa, and attended Elgin Community College in Illinois. She works as an ortho/spine nurse clinician for a large, private orthopedic practice in Geneva, Illinois. In addition, Cary is attending the University of Phoenix on-line in pursuit of her BSN. She is newly remarried and has a 19-year-old son who is a freshman in college. They have a houseful of pets: three small birds, four parrots, and two dogs. She can be reached at Birdijo@aol.com.

Work*able* Wisdom

- **Remember you are forging a path for others.** People with disabilities have not been welcomed with open arms into nursing. We must work extra hard and be extra competent, just like any other minority does when trying to pave the trail for others to follow.

- **Don't ever use your problems as an excuse for not doing your job properly.** Consider this example: "I was tired, so I didn't pass the meds." Find a way to get the job done, even if it's asking for help. If you have a disability, you have a label. Don't let that label be associated with a difficult working situation for others, or they will not welcome those who follow. Who wants to work with a bipolar nurse when the one they worked with last was a flake who never assessed patients thoroughly?

- **Do not ask for accommodations unless you really need them.** This will earn you and others like you respect from coworkers, instead of groaning when your name is on the schedule.

- **Take care of yourself.** If you have a chronic condition like diabetes, don't forget to carry snacks and eat meals when indicated.

- **Be professional.** Do not take care of patients even for one hour if you are mentally incapable of doing so competently. Patient safety must always come first. If you are not all there mentally for any reason, do not report for work.

- **Remind your hospital administrators that you're a knowledgeable worker.** A nurse with 25 years of ICU experience and excellent critical thinking skills should not be tossed aside as soon as she has a bad back. This just doesn't make sense. These experienced nurses with disabilities are leaders, mentors and the backbone of any unit.

6

Setting Sun: Nursing with Retinitis Pigmentosis

By Mary Tozzo, RN, MS

When I was old enough to be allowed to play outside after dinner, I was always the first to retreat back home. The enveloping darkness left me unable to see what the other children could. Little did I know that the darkness was enveloping me in more ways than one.

After my persistent complaining, my mother took me to a doctor. But he told my mother that there was nothing wrong with my eyes—that I was simply trying to get attention. He advised her to ignore my behavior.

As I got older, I knew that I had more accidents than the average child. I stepped or tripped over objects that others easily avoided. I was often bruised and believed that I must just be an uncoordinated klutz. I was always the last picked for sports and dreaded any event that required coordination. I assumed that I just didn't have the best reflexes. Because I did not fit in with the other children, I buried myself in books.

By the time I was a senior in high school, I found that I could competently participate in activities such as writing for and editing the school newspaper, chairing events such as the Toys-for-Tots campaign and delivering oratory presentations at competitions. I was in the national honor society and was the headline speaker at my hometown's "I am an American" night, where new citizens were sworn in. I boldly decided that I wanted to become a nurse and began sending for college catalogs. The future seemed so full of possibilities.

My dad pointed out that night classes might be difficult for me because of my inability to see after dark. Despite the doctor's declaration that there was no medical basis for my complaints, my father unconditionally believed me from the start.

My mother made another appointment for me with the same eye doctor I had seen previously. Luckily, he was very busy that day, and I was deferred to his younger partner. That doctor listened to my experiences, reviewed my chart and examined my eyes. I still remember how numb I felt when he told me that I had retinitis pigmentosa. He explained that it was a progressive disease that would eventually result in complete blindness.

It usually does not become apparent in someone as young as I was at that time. But because I was born prematurely, I was placed in 100% oxygen at birth. That had accelerated the disease process.

This doctor seemed surprised that the diagnosis had been missed. I had been reporting all of the textbook symptoms. I was taken to a well-known hospital for days of testing. The diagnosis was confirmed. The specialists declared that I was already legally blind and predicted that I would probably become totally blind sometime between the ages of 30 and 50.

I was asked what career path I had chosen. Every doctor vehemently shook his head "no" when I said I wanted to become a nurse. They all agreed that I had lost too much vision to be able to perform such a job. Worrying about being able to perform the job was a moot point anyway, since I would never be able to do the reading required to earn a BSN degree in the first place, they said.

My head spun as I returned home. I cannot say what I did over the next few weeks. I managed to get up in the morning and go to school, but I went through those weeks in a fog. I had been diagnosed with diabetes at age 10 and had already been told to expect that to create complications in the future. This seemed like the final straw for me.

My mother felt guilty for not believing my reports of vision problems and was determined to find me a miracle. We embarked on a family tour of the shrines in Canada in search of her miracle. I had always believed that God was by your side—no matter where you were. But I agreed to go on the trip anyway to appease her. It was a unique experience, but we returned without the quick fix my mother had hoped for.

The time in Canada allowed me time to reflect on what I wanted to do with my life and what I had to do to achieve it. I decided to ignore the doctors' warnings and give college a try. After all, you cannot go anywhere if you don't take the first step. I also have this stubborn streak that makes me want to try even harder when told that something can't be done. I'd rather say that someone just hasn't figured out how to do something yet.

I enrolled in a four-year nursing program in a neighboring state, despite my family's insistence that I attend school closer to home. I got back in the swing of my senior year and applied myself to my studies as diligently as I had in the past. I won the "Family Leader of Tomorrow" award and was inducted into the Society of Distinguished American High School Students. At graduation, I was presented with a trophy for excellence in English and chemistry and another for general excellence in college preparatory subjects.

Although I had adjusted to the everyday problems my visual loss had imposed, I still remember fearing my graduation ceremony. It was to be held in an old church that was dimly lit. My teacher, Sister Rose, was kind enough to arrange for all students to be escorted to the podium to receive their awards and diplomas. That way I would not stand out. I don't know if she understood how much that meant to me.

College came with its own challenges. During the day, I walked where I could and took the bus to places I couldn't walk to. I used flashlights to travel to classes in nearby buildings at night. Luckily, it was not a large campus, and I managed by just taking my time and using landmarks to ensure that I was going in the right direction. I researched aids for the visually impaired and asked my counselor at the division of the blind to purchase a night scope for me. Initially, he wanted to decline my request. They had never purchased one before. But I pushed him. My request was eventually approved, giving me greater freedom to walk without human assistance at night. I was also blessed to have understanding friends who helped transport me to clinical settings and other places that were farther away from campus or inaccessible by bus.

I attended mixers and joined my friends at the local watering holes, grateful for their assistance. We used my visual handicap for practical jokes at times. On one night, I went out with a male friend to the local mall. He had been strictly told by several of our friends that he was not to leave me anywhere alone. When we returned to the dorm, I hid and he proceeded to inform them, in a panic, that he lost me. After the initial melee, we revealed our prank, and everyone had a good laugh.

In some instances, I had to level the playing field myself. Once a friend started a snowball fight in a parking lot at night, where I could not see. I finished the fight in his car, where I could see. I was declared the winner.

Back in the '70s, when I was in college, you were on your own when it came to getting disability accommodations. At times, it was difficult to complete the required readings left on hold in the library, as my eyes tired easily. I compensated by photocopying the material and taking them back to the dorm, where I could read at my own pace. I'm sure that over the years I pumped enough money into that copy machine to build a second library.

Only one instructor felt that my visual handicap required intervention, but it was not something that I desired. She offered to let me forgo reading assignments that were required of others. I politely declined. I wanted to know that I received a grade because I had earned it and not because she felt sorry for me.

In another instance, an instructor did not believe that I was visually impaired. She accused me of cheating on a quiz. I was shocked, as I would rather flunk than even consider cheating. I tried to explain that I was legally blind and did not have enough vision to cheat if I had wanted to. I told her that I would have to be sitting *in* someone's lap in order to be able to read their work clearly enough to cheat off their paper

Despite the obstacles, I graduated with a bachelor's degree in nursing with a near-perfect grade point average. I was inducted into the National Dean's List and Who's Who Among Students in American Universities and Colleges. I also published a poem in the American Collegiate Poet's Anthology.

My first job after graduation was in the state where I attended college. Again, my family wanted me to work closer to home. But I wanted to try to make it on my own. Besides, I had the security of knowing that I could always go home if I did not succeed.

I secured a job in a hospital on a 20-bed oncology unit. I had always enjoyed teaching and asked to be placed on a unit that had diabetic patients, so that I could ease myself into diabetes education. I was told that the unit that housed diabetic patients was sufficiently staffed, so I was being placed on the next unit over. They didn't mention that it was the oncology unit, as most nurses then refused the assignment.

But I found that I enjoyed working with these patients. I got to know many of them and their families as closely as if they were members of my own family. Other nurses asked me how I could be part of such a depressing area of practice. I found it to be a wonderfully enriching experience.

At this point, my visual limitations interfered with only a few aspects of my job. I had difficulty in dim or dark hallways or rooms. I required another nurse to examine pupils during neurological checks. I had been working there only a few months when the RN who held the charge position on one of the shifts resigned. I was designated to assume the position. I was the youngest and the newest nurse to ever hold the position. I was lucky to be working with several seasoned LPNs who mentored me.

During that time, I met someone and got married. After two years, we decided that it was time for a move. My husband liked Florida. We first visited during a vacation. I interviewed at multiple hospitals before accepting a position at a small hospital on a three-wing, 68-bed unit. I was to start my new job just one week after the move. Then unexpectedly I received a telegram informing me that I would not be allowed to start as scheduled.

I phoned human resources and was told that the decision had been made by the chief nursing officer. I called the chief nursing officer, but she would not give me a reason for the delay. I demanded a meeting. I had just moved 1,500 miles to accept this job. When I arrived for the meeting, I was told that my medical records had arrived. After reviewing them, she felt that I would not be capable of performing my job as a bedside nurse, even though I had already been interviewed by the unit's nurse manager and had been hired on the spot. I asked how she could judge a person based on medical records alone. In my previous job, I had not only been in charge of the floor, but I simultaneously carried a patient as well. When I pointed that out to her, she said she thought I only handled desk duties. In the end, she allowed me to start as scheduled.

At first, there was a palpable resentment among the nurses. They had been forewarned that I was visually impaired. They feared that they would have to "carry" a handicapped nurse. I had to prove myself. I had to give 150% to receive credit for 50%.

After seven years of marriage, my husband and I divorced. It was time again to reassess my life. My friends and family assumed that I could return to the safety of my roots. My dad offered to let me move back home. He said that he would be willing to drive me to and from work if it was needed. But I decided to try to stick it out on my own. It was terrifying.

I worked many double shifts in order to keep the home that I loved. When I did begin dating, it was extremely challenging. Since I can make eye contact, it is not always obvious that I am visually impaired. It's difficult to casually slip into the conversation that you are legally blind. I allowed friends to fix me up without success. After all, I gave true meaning to the phrase "blind date." I even tried my luck at the personals. At first I just listened to the recorded messages before hanging up. Eventually, I got the nerve up to answer a few ads. That was quite an experience. I found that most men my age had been married, had families, gotten divorced and were ready to start a second family.

During my marriage, I'd had two miscarriages and a stillborn child at full term. I was not looking for someone who wanted additional children. I met a wide variety of people, but no sparks flew. I eventually met an engineer. We compared dating horror stories. He later admitted that he could tell that something was off when we met, but he did not realize what until I later admitted that I was visually impaired.

We had a good laugh over one date that almost happened with another personal ad suitor. I had talked on the phone with this gentleman several times, but we had not met in person yet. He proposed to take me to a local fair one evening. I commented that since it would dark out, I would need to hang onto his arm because of my poor vision. "Well, it's not like you're legally blind or anything, is it?" he responded. I waited a couple of beats and then said, "Yeah. As a matter of fact, I am." There was dead silence on the other end of the phone. We never did go out.

A defining moment occurred with the engineer one evening when he came over for a date. I had handed him a bottle of non-alcoholic beer, and we began talking. He had only taken one sip when I extended my arm to make a point and accidentally knocked the bottle clean out of his hand. It hit the ceramic tile like a bomb. I stiffened. My ex-husband used to yell at me when I knocked over or broke something. I waited for the usual tirade. We stood in silence.

Finally he said, "Well..."

"Well what?" I asked, half afraid.

"Aren't you going to yell at me?" he said. Imagine my surprise.

"I thought you were going to yell at me!" I exclaimed.

"Are you hurt?" he asked.

"No. Are you hurt?" I replied.

"No," he said. "Finally, a woman who doesn't overreact over something insignificant." We were both relieved.

I did eventually prove myself at work, to the point where I was awarded the hospital's Nurse of the Year award. I was presented with two tickets to San Francisco, where my present husband proposed. I have worked at that same hospital for the last 20 years.

In that time, I have seen a lot of changes in the profession and healthcare in general. Bedside nursing has become a treacherous balancing act, where nurses are required to be traffic cops capable of managing the needs of patients, doctors, family members and administrators. Patients that used to be in ICU are now part of a typical assignment. Nurses must also oversee others in ancillary departments, ensuring that the correct medications have arrived from the pharmacy and have been properly dispensed, that labs have been drawn, and that diagnostic tests have been performed. Those aspects are a cakewalk for me.

Unfortunately, nurses today must also complete reams of paperwork and manage multiple pieces of complex medical equipment. As my vision dimmed, my comfort with bedside nursing waned. I begged to be placed in an education position where my failing vision would not cause me as much discomfort.

Despite the fact that I earned certification in all three areas of specialty on the unit (as a med-surg nurse and oncology nurse clinician, and a certified diabetes educator), I was still serving primarily as a bedside nurse. But it became increasingly difficult to perform these duties without patients picking up on my impairment. Patients and visitors have made disparaging comments at times that I have tried to attribute to ignorance. But they hurt no less.

Lighting in our hospital rooms has changed over the years. We now have energy-saving fixtures and wall switches are now located at the center of the rooms' back walls, requiring one to stumble through the dark and over multiple obstacles to find the switch. More forms with increasing items requiring documentation have been added to nurses' daily list of tasks, and the print on these forms has shrunk. First it was the medication administration record, then the admission assessment form and lastly the nurses' daily notes and assessment forms.

The medical equipment that the hospital chose to use, including feeding, intravenous and patient-controlled analgesia pumps, as well as blood glucose monitors, have screens with displays that I cannot read. I didn't like having to ask others to do my job for me, so I began to feel as if I was no longer able to meet my own expectations for myself. I became determined to work my way into the educational aspect of nursing.

Seven years ago, I enrolled in graduate school. This event was precipitated by my acquaintance with a dynamite counselor from the Division of Blind Services. He introduced me to the National Federation of the Blind, where I met many individuals who were functioning as doctors, lawyers, teachers, etc., despite being completely blind. I was petrified of going back to school, but I knew that if they could do it, so could I. My counselor promised to do all he could to help me reach my goal.

I was surprised to find that some schools had a disability services office, and they provided accommodations for people like me. They offered note takers and enlarged the print on my tests. The first class I was required to take was statistics, or sadistics, as I not-so-fondly called it. I found that I could not read the board, so I asked for a note taker. This turned out to be quite an ordeal. Volunteers were hard to find. Despite the fact that I took my own notes on whatever information was presented verbally and only needed someone to write down the equations, no note taker lasted for more than three weeks. One had the gall to attend only two classes and then charge for seven.

The professor had been told before the start of the semester that he would need to provide me with hardcopies of anything that he presented on the board or as a visual aide. Nothing was ever provided. He wrote on the board during every class. He'd look at me and ask, "Do you see?" I would have to repeat that no, my vision had not mysteriously returned since the last class. During the third class I found out that we would be using a statistics program on the computer. I was the oldest student in the class—everyone else was fresh out of high school—and I had never used a personal computer. Everyone else was on the seventh screen while I was still trying to find the on button. There I was, trying to learn how to use a computer and learn statistics at the same time.

The screen and keyboard were a strain to read. Thankfully, my counselor came to the rescue with a large monitor and keyboard with oversized print overlays installed in the classroom. Overall, I think my guide dog summed up my feelings about that class the best—she threw up on the carpet in the classroom the first day of class.

Throughout the years, the Office of Disability Services adapted their accommodations to my declining vision. I was able to read most of my textbooks with magnifiers until the last year. When that became too difficult, the DS office enlarged my texts on a photocopier.

It was a long road, with more adaptations along the way, including a larger computer monitor at home and the installation of Zoomtext. I frequently wondered why I was putting myself through this ordeal. The only saving grace was a very supportive husband who did his best to keep things in perspective, although he spent seven years in fear that one day my frustration would get the better of me and in one good heave I'd teach the computer to fly.

I am thrilled to say that I graduated with my master's in nursing education with a 4.0 GPA. I don't know whose smile is bigger in the graduation photo—my guide dog's or mine. She knew something special was going on when the entire audience gave us a standing ovation as we crossed the stage to receive our degree.

I now work as a clinical educator, teaching nursing orientation and presenting continuing education classes. I created a certified nursing assistant skills orientation program and am the designated certified diabetes educator for the facility. I provide both inpatient and outpatient diabetes education. I have yet to shake the charge role and act as relief charge nurse when needed and on every other weekend. I have maintained certification in all three specialty areas on the unit and am the most credentialed nurse in the hospital.

The certification agencies have always provided large print exams, although the answer sheets have not been adaptable. They have, however, offered to have someone fill in the circles for me as I take exams. Studying for the tests has become more difficult, as I must enlarge all of my study materials. It is worth it though. I like to constantly challenge myself.

Others tell me that there are things that a legally blind person should not attempt, but I still give some a try. One of those was hang-gliding in Mexico. I still remember the look on the instructor's face. He told me he'd signal me in to land with his arms and I told him that I would not be able to see him because I was legally blind. He stressed that I must land on the beach, near the water's edge. I had visions of landing on one of the tiki huts, speared like a shish kabob. Despite my disability, I was the only person who landed where I was supposed. Others had to be rescued by boat from deep in the water.

I have learned from my patients that life is a precious gift and that we should appreciate every moment of it, being thankful for what we have rather than lamenting what we don't. My father taught me to stand my ground and fight those fights I deem worth fighting for. I live my life by a creed from an anonymous author that I found after my diagnosis in my senior year of high school. It states, "I am only one, but I am one. I cannot do everything, but I can do something. What I can do, I ought to do. And what I ought to do, by the grace of God, I will do."

Mary Tozzo, RN, MS, is clinical nurse educator who teaches orientation and continuing education classes at a hospital in south Florida. She is the designated certified diabetes educator for the facility and provides both inpatient and outpatient diabetes education. Mary received her master's degree in nursing from Barry University. She lives with her husband and guide dog in south Florida.

Work*able* Wisdom

- **Take chances.** Whether it's going back to school or hang-gliding, don't let a disability hold you back. You will never know if you can do something if you don't at least try.

- **Don't get discouraged by an inconsiderate professor or tough class.** When it comes to progressive disabilities, preparing for the future is key to making sure you can continue to work in the field as a condition worsens. And preparing often means going back to college. While you may certainly encounter unsupportive professors, don't let them keep you from the future you want for yourself.

- **Do what you must to prove yourself.** It is an unfortunate reality that nurses with disabilities must work twice as hard as others to prove their competence on the job. But if you do that early, you will soon gain the trust and respect of your coworkers—and you will make it easier for other nurses with disabilities to do the same.

7

Shake, Rattle and Roll: Nursing with Fine Motor Tremor, Depression and Cancer

By Nicole Freeman, RN, BSN

I was about 13, working as a candy striper at a local nursing home in Syracuse, New York, when I decided that I wanted to be a nurse. Working with two doctors had a lot to do with my decision. One doctor had very sloppy penmanship, so I wrote his standing orders while he watched, and then he signed them. An ophthalmologist also came to the nursing home monthly to run an eye clinic. I transported his patients from their rooms to the clinic in the basement of the nursing home.

I enjoyed working with both of the physicians. They were both semi-retired, very pleasant, and enjoyed teaching. Dr. Frank, the eye doctor, took great delight in telling me stories of eye surgeries and how neurosurgery nurses "can handle seeing brains all the time, but do a simple eye operation with me, and see one eye ball, and they're done."

I also enjoyed the one-on-one contact with clients—even the disagreeable ones who would spit at me or hurl their scrambled eggs. I liked to hang out with my friend Nellie. She was blind, 93 years-old and talked my ear off. I did manicures for Helen, whose gnarled hands and thick, yellow nails belied her 160-pack-a year-smoking history.

When I worked with the doctors, we spent less than 10 minutes in each room. The clients barely had time to say "hello." The science of medicine was interesting, but I noticed it was actually the nurses who were there with the patients—all the time. They held people's hands, soothed confused minds, passed meds, talked to patients, and even on horribly hectic days found time to do the little extras that mattered so much to patients.

In high school, my desire for a career in medicine or nursing grew. I had originally wanted to be a veterinarian, but I became allergic to all animals with fur, so that was out. I spent a year in a medical explorer's post, learning more about healthcare professions. In 1978, I entered a three-year registered nursing program at the Crouse Irving Hospital School of Nursing, and I finished in 1981.

During my first year as a registered nurse, I learned to be a charge nurse, rotate all three shifts in the same week and juggle large numbers of patients. I also learned how to go long hours without meals or bathroom breaks.

My father retired to Utah in 1982. I moved there with my parents and to get away from my allergy problems and the miserable central New York climate. At that point in my career, I wanted to try critical care nursing. I recall getting a slight indication that I had trouble with my hands around this time. When I was under a great deal of stress, or nervous, they shook. I figured it was something everyone's hands did.

I found my first critical care job at the University of Utah in 1982. I learned the art of medical and coronary intensive nursing and was amazed and continually challenged by the variety of patients and problems I encountered there. I met amazing nurses, physicians and patients. There was an atmosphere of constant learning.

I was in my early 20s then and was able to handle the stress of working 12-hour night shifts on a short-staffed unit with high turnover. We had four nurse managers in two years.

I looked out the window of the ICU and saw the helicopters coming in and out and thought, "I can do that some day." I had burned out on ICU, so I moved to the emergency department—and one step closer to the flight team. I became part of the ED staff and got busy getting certifications: advanced cardiac life support, basic cardiac life support, burn trauma life support and certified emergency nursing. I also started teaching resuscitation classes and working with some of the emergency medical technician and paramedic students.

During that time, I developed an orientation program for RNs. I continued to work full-time in the ED until 1989, soaking up whatever I could in terms of the science of medicine and nursing. When the attending physicians talked to the residents and interns, I listened. I picked the brains of nurses with whom I worked.

Then, I met my future husband. On our first date, I spilled my tea. I have always been a little clumsy. In retrospect, he also wonders if that was part of the little "disconnect" that went with my tremor. I was always spilling things.

I secured a part-time position with the flight team in 1988 and went full-time in 1989. I flew in helicopters and airplanes, covering a seven-state area. It was a fascinating job that often took me from the desert to the alpines within an hour. I sometimes ended up in odd places that I would otherwise not likely find on a map.

It was the summer of 1990 and everything seemed perfect. I was in a steady relationship on the verge of marriage, successful in my job and generally just loving life. Then disaster struck. I experienced my first bout of mental illness.

I took a five-month leave of absence from work because of severe clinical depression. I tried multiple antidepressants before finding the correct combination. I have the misfortune of being very sensitive to many medications and their side effects.

A self-help group for people with depression called Recovery, Inc., was instrumental in my recovery. It consists of cognitive therapy. A book by the group's founder, *Mental Health Through Will Training*, helped me regain and maintain my mental health. With the right combination of medication, a good psychiatrist, Recovery, Inc., and my family and fiancé, I was soon able to go back to work. My employer was patient and worked with me by allowing me to work half time. They made me feel valued and gave me something to look forward to. (See Appendix A, Sample Accommodation Request Letter.)

Jeff and I got married on Christmas Eve of 1990. Shortly after, Jeff shipped out to Desert Storm. While he was gone, I worked with the flight team and continued my recovery. When he returned, we set up our household and adjusted to married life. Things were relatively quiet for about two years.

Then, over the course of a weekend, I became ill with what I thought was appendicitis or the flu. Three days later, I was hospitalized with what was ultimately diagnosed as a malignant renal cell carcinoma of the right kidney. It required a radical nephrectomy and lymph node dissection. I had not required chemotherapy or radiation.

After a seven-week leave of absence, I was able to return to work. Life with one kidney proved to be more or less the same as with two. But I was not as ready to work as I thought, and the first few days I crawled home after each shift. Mentally, it was very difficult to adjust to having cancer.

For many weeks and months, it seemed that I was assigned every last patient with terminal renal cell carcinoma in the western states. I was preoccupied with morbid thoughts. I had a great deal of difficulty thinking ahead and making plans for the future. It was the first time I had come face-to-face with my own mortality. The enormous scar was there every day as a reminder, and I investigated every backache and muscle cramp that I would have previously dismissed.

One day, I was nearly hit by a car while going to see my oncologist. The incident "snapped my garters." It finally occurred to me that you could live your life waiting for cancer to return, or you could move on with your life and make it very difficult for the cancer to find you again. This is not to say that I don't become alarmed any time my renal functions are tested or a backache lasts too long. But I decided to keep living. I went on to have two children. My first delivery was difficult, but all my symptoms resolved themselves after I gave birth. I continued to work as an emergency nurse in Rockford, Illinois.

In April 1999, my father died of an advanced abdominal tumor that was not diagnosed until three weeks prior to his death. I was pregnant with my daughter at the time and shuttling back and forth between Utah and Illinois for months before he died. I managed his health problems and ran interference with his physicians. I essentially became his case manager. Our experiences with his medical care left me feeling betrayed by the healthcare industry. The indifferent care he received required that my family and I constantly nag and check up on every aspect of his care, right down to telling the physician what meds to order when he went home in hospice.

My daughter was born in October of that same year, and although the pregnancy was uneventful, I was hypertensive in the weeks following delivery. Towards January of 2000, I noticed that as I nursed my daughter, my right arm and shoulder sometimes felt numb, tingly and at times even shaky. It always went away, so I continued to ignore it.

Three months after my daughter was born, I went to work again as a flight nurse. In retrospect, going back to working full-time was a mistake. My stress level shot up, as the job was very demanding. The unit was in transition at the time, and the duties of the flight crew were in flux. In addition, I was rotating shifts and not getting enough sleep. The tremor reappeared. I had been trying to do way too much.

One day, while practicing airway management with an anesthesiologist in the operating suite, my right hand and arm began shaking uncontrollably as I placed an airway. "You need more practice. What's the matter with you?" he snapped. I had no idea what had happened. I thought it was the two cups of coffee that I'd had while waiting for him. The tremor went away as soon as the anesthesiologist did. I continued to work. I was shaken up, of course, but I didn't seek care.

That summer, I felt a sense of unease growing inside me. My hands shook more often. The right hand was worse. It shook when I was under pressure, especially when rushing to do something like getting medications drawn up swiftly. I felt anxious quite often and had a great deal of difficulty sleeping. I realized that I could stay awake for 24 hours straight. And I began to notice a nearly continuous fine tremor in both hands. My writing deteriorated, and when I was triaging, my charting worsened. I would start a sentence, and within three or four words, the letters were indistinguishable.

Finally, I went to my family practice physician and began taking Mysoline for the tremors. But I had fallen back into depression. I felt fearful all the time, and I had nightmares and acid reflux. And I was irritable. Life seemed to accelerate faster and faster. As I unconsciously turned inward more, I developed a constant preoccupation with the possibility of developing a permanent condition.

In late September 2000, over the course of a couple of days, everything finally caved in. It felt like a great black bird—a giant pterodactyl perhaps—had settled over my house, casting its dark presence over everything. By October, I started a leave of absence from work and began taking antidepressants. I saw a local neurologist who conclusively ruled out multiple sclerosis. When I had exhausted my sick leave and vacation days, I went on short-term disability.

I saw an excellent psychiatrist, who worked and reworked the medication regimen to try to find some combination that treated the depression and obsessive thinking and did not aggravate the tremor. But there were setbacks. Lithium caused a significant worsening of the tremor. It got to the point that I could barely walk or feed myself.

By January 2001, I had quit my job entirely. It became apparent that the essential tremor was permanent and could not be sufficiently controlled so as to allow me to perform the required fine motor skills.

Had I stayed in Illinois, my previous employers said they would have tried to find something that I could do, but otherwise they offered very little. They did not offer any suggestions or assistance concerning long-term disability. Luckily, my husband received a significant promotion within his company. It required that we moved to Colorado, so we packed up and went.

We agreed that I would not work outside the home while I finished my BSN. That way, I could concentrate on my education. I enrolled at Regis University. I was determined to finish the degree that I had been chipping away at for the past 15 years. I also began formulating a plan. I knew that my fine motor skills were probably going to be permanently impaired. I decided to put my disability to work for me, looking at a broad spectrum of opportunities within the field of nursing. As I turned towards the things that I could do, I realized that I was still an intelligent, thoughtful, resourceful and creative individual—my hands just didn't work very well. As a nurse with more than two decades of experience, I knew that I had a lot to offer.

When I enrolled at Regis University, the first thing I did was swallow my pride and go to the institution's disabilities access Web page. I realized that I would not be able to keep up with note taking in classes, and I was going to have difficulties with extensive writing. I explored what was required to obtain accommodations. An admissions counselor verified with the nursing department that they could accommodate my specific needs. My doctor supplied the necessary documentation. The school provided me with a note taker, free double-page notepaper, extra time during tests, computer testing and oral exams. I also asked for and received installation of DragonSpeak—a voice recognition software program that obviates the need for manual key boarding—on university computers on two campuses. This enhanced my ability to take tests and write papers at school.

It is possible to get more or different accommodations if a disability requires it, as long as such requests are supported by documentation and they are reasonable. A student cannot, for example, request an accommodation that would give him an unreasonable advantage.

I was required to give each instructor a form letter that detailed what accommodations I required. I also kept a copy. The instructor or I could ask for a volunteer note taker. The instructor and the note taker were required to keep the nature of my disability confidential. However, mine was pretty obvious.

I was uncomfortable accepting help with writing and carrying drinks and embarrassed when I dropped things, spilled drinks and so on. But I realized that most people got over their initial curiosity very quickly. If they asked a question, I gave them simple, straightforward answers. They were satisfied and accepted me as readily as any other student. Student peers, as a rule, tend to be generous about offering assistance, whether it be with opening things, taking notes or any of the other frustrating fine motor tasks that come up. More than one note taker had to be convinced to take the stipend from the disabilities office, as opposed to doing the notes for free.

Another example of the willingness of the school and its staff to accommodate me stands out in my mind. One professor had allowed me to go to the computer lab to complete an essay test. I felt particularly shaky that day, so I used the computer with the DragonSpeak voice recognition software. Suddenly, in the middle of the exam, the entire system crashed. I lost my test. When I finally recovered my document, time for the test was nearly over, and I was barely one-third of the way done. My frustration with the computer worsened my tremor, which always intensified with heightened emotion. I rushed back to class and asked if I could test in another venue. He readily agreed, even though he was not really prepared to do so. I was able to finish the test that way.

At home, I often use Dragon NaturallySpeaking voice recognition program to surf the Internet, write e-mail, and compose my papers. It usually saves me about three hours of writing for every hour that I actually spend dictating. The software creates a voice file unique to each user. The more you use it, the more it learns and the more accurate it becomes at recognizing your words. The version I use readily acquired healthcare-related words. When I do manual typing, I generally work with my left hand. When I do a presentation, I put my right hand in my pocket, as it is usually the worst offender. Also, I use yoga breathing techniques for relaxation before presenting in public. I find these little tricks helpful because my tremors are always worse in situations such as public speaking, when my anxiety levels spike.

I graduated from the RN to BSN program at Regis University at the end of 2003. What the future holds for me in nursing, I am not certain. However, I have achieved my long-held goal, despite a significant disability and while raising my two children. In the process, I have overcome my health issues. I would like to go on to graduate school, with the ultimate goal of teaching or writing. While I may be away from the bedside, I have never wanted to stop giving back to others—what nurses do every day.

I found a neurologist who was finally able to find a better medication solution for my tremors. I applied for a job with a company called Care Core National, which pre-approves radiological procedures for health insurance companies. At the interviews, I came right out about my handicap.

I was hired for the position and was fortunate that the company accommodated my needs by purchasing an adaptive mouse developed by IBM. Also, I was given special permission to do all my typing in capital letters to improve my one-handed typing. In addition, the technical support personnel work with me to help me improve my computing abilities.

I volunteer at a program in Colorado Springs that provides free healthcare and health counseling to the homeless and underserved. I enjoy the contact with the community of clients that we serve. While I do miss the excitement and intensity of flight, emergency and critical care nursing, I recognize that this disability has sent my life and career in directions that I may not otherwise have explored. It has made it possible for me to show others that as a nurse, I am far more than a pair of hands, disability or no disability.

Nicole Freeman, RN, BSN, is the married mother of two children. She graduated from a diploma program in Syracuse, New York. Later, she received a BSN from Regis University. Since 1981, Nicole has worked as an intensive care nurse, emergency nurse and flight nurse. She developed essential and Parkinsonian tremors. The tremor affects all of her limbs, especially her dominant hand. She has also overcome kidney cancer. Nicole currently works for Care Core National. She can be reached at nlf5cents@adelphia.net.

Work*able* Wisdom

- **Put your pride aside to put yourself before your disability.** Seeking disability accommodations can seem like admitting defeat. But often accommodation is what it takes to conquer your disability and move on with your life.

- **Realize that you can still contribute.** You may not be able to continue working as a critical care nurse—or in Nicole's situation, as a flight nurse. But that doesn't mean you still don't have a lot to offer the nursing profession. Figure out what you can do instead of dwelling on what you can't.

- **Be up front about your disability.** If you're not up front, you will leave people wondering, particularly if your disability is clearly visible. And if people—professors, employer or coworkers—don't know what exactly effects your disability has on you, they might be prone to think you are capable of less than you are.

◆   ◆   ◆

Low, A. (1997). *Mental health through will training* (3rd edition). Glencoe, IL: Willett Pub.

8

The Little Engine That Could: Nursing with Profound Deafness

By Morag MacDonald, RN, MSW

I was born in Belleville, Ontario, in 1957, the first-generation daughter of a Scottish mother and English father. My two older sisters were born in England, and my younger brother was born in Canada. At birth, I was diagnosed with a congenital heart defect secondary to an ototoxic medication that my mother took during the first trimester of her pregnancy.

At 6 weeks of age, I was also diagnosed with severe, progressive hearing loss. I am now profoundly deaf. My younger brother also sustained severe to profound hearing loss due to an infection he acquired at 20 months of age and cytomegalovirus, which my mother contracted during pregnancy.

I was raised within the pathological view often held by society in general that a hearing loss is something that must be fixed. When individuals identify themselves as being a Deaf person with a capital "D," it shows cultural pride, whereas use of the word with a lower case "d" denotes the pathological view. This differentiation will be important as you read more about my life.

I was taught to read lips and speak. My mother knew early on that I was deaf because I did not respond to sounds like my two older sisters had. She began to hold me upright, facing her, instead of along the side of her body. That way, I was constantly facing her. She talked and sang to me as if I were a hearing baby. I believe this was why, lacking audiological training, I developed speech at an unusually early age for a person with severe hearing loss. "Once she started talking, she never stopped!" my mother used to say about me.

Whether she realized it or not, my mother maintained the pathological view and trained me to function in the dominant hearing society. Traditionally, many d/Deaf people lack incidental learning experiences due to their inability to absorb information through casual conversations, such as family table talk, radio, television and other daily interaction with the world. I was curious about the world around me and constantly asked questions. My mother would stop whatever she was doing and take the time to explain things to me. I was also fortunate that my family had a deep love for reading that was passed on to me.

I first learned that I was different when I was 4 years old. I was hospitalized for seven weeks due to my congenital heart defect, which was repaired successfully. While I was in the hospital, I shared a room with three other girls. I noticed that the other children did not have to look at each other to talk and play. It was the first time that I felt left out of the world around me.

Parents were not allowed to remain in the hospital with their children at that time. I became curious about the things going on around me. I asked the nurses a lot of questions about what they did. This was my earliest introduction to the healthcare culture. My doctor even told my mother that I was a nurse in the making. I decided at that time that I was going to be a nurse. But I learned that people were skeptical—condescending even—about the idea of me wanting to become a nurse.

My family had immigrated to the United States when I was almost 3 years old. My father had been offered a better job opportunity. Shortly after moving to Long Island, I was enrolled in a school for the Deaf, where lip-reading and speech were emphasized. Despite that, I felt there a sense of belonging there because I was with other children like me.

I remained at the school for the Deaf until the age of 10, when my family moved to Massachusetts. There, I became the school's poster child, representing it at numerous fundraisers to demonstrate how d/Deaf people can be taught to lip-read and speak. These events increased my confidence in public speaking.

I transitioned to a local public school, which I attended from the fifth to tenth grade without any support services, such as interpreters or note takers. I basically had no natural incidental learning experiences in the classroom during those years. I was regarded by most teachers as the "poor deaf girl." I learned almost exclusively through books. I transferred to a college preparatory school for the last two years of high school. It was there that I got the most support and encouragement to pursue my dream of becoming a nurse.

Applying to nursing school was a challenge. It was the first time I remember feeling as if I was being slapped in the face for wanting to chase my dream. On the advice of my guidance counselor, I applied to two colleges as a nursing major. I also applied to two schools as a special education major, with the idea that I could later switch to a nursing major if I got accepted into the education program. I was accepted into the two special education programs and rejected by the two nursing programs.

During my high school and college years, I worked as a nurse's aide at a group home and a nursing home for the severely mentally retarded. I also worked for three years as a personal care assistant for three quadriplegic students at my college. Caring for people who were different from me was a shaping experience. It also sensitized me to the challenges faced by people who may not be able to verbally communicate their needs.

I learned sign language when I met my roommate at the preparatory school. It was through her that I found a job at a camp in Martha's Vineyard for children with multiple disabilities. I held the job for three summers. During that time, I began to appreciate myself as a Deaf person. I felt fortunate to have the abilities to lip-read, speak well and communicate fluently in sign language.

I became further exposed to Deaf Culture during my freshman year at the University of Massachusetts at Amherst. There, I began socializing with Deaf students on campus. I was only involved with the dominant hearing culture during class times, work and sorority life. The rest of my time was spent with my Deaf friends, interpreters and sign language students.

I switched my major to nursing. Then, due to poor grades, I was asked to leave the program. But I became determined to work harder and regain entry into the nursing program by continuing the courses necessary for a nursing degree. Unfortunately, the university decided to close its nursing school at the end of my freshman year. When in the middle of my sophomore year it reopened, I reapplied. My grades had improved, so I thought I'd have no problem getting into the program. Here I encountered discrimination.

I had to go through a "pathological" admission process different from that of the hearing applicants. I had to obtain proof that a person with my kind of deafness, now profoundly Deaf, could succeed as a nurse. I also had to undergo more interviews with various faculty members than did my hearing peers. I was accepted on a "conditional basis," meaning if there were no problems with my performance or grades, the following year I would be considered fully admitted.

Reapplying to nursing school taught me the importance of asserting myself to get what I wanted. I had to persuade others that my Deafness was not a barrier. I graduated from the School of Nursing in 1980 with honors. Helping me get through my coursework were the use of an amplified stethoscope, a frequency modulated amplification system for clinical experiences, and interpreters and note takers for class.

I learned quickly during my clinical rotations with patients not to use the word "Deaf" when identifying myself. Doing so often triggered an automatic pathological reaction from the patient that someone defective could not be an effective caregiver. I found that the label "hearing impaired" put the patients at ease more then the term "Deaf." I feel that "hearing impaired" is a generic and sometimes confusing term. It covers all kinds and degrees of hearing loss. It can be used as a safety net or to hide how grave the hearing loss is. Nowadays, it is a relief not to have to identify myself as "hearing impaired," since I now work for Deaf and Hard-of-Hearing Services. Now, I do not have to give up my self-identity as a Deaf nurse to reassure my patients of my competence as a caregiver.

My first job as a nurse was on the spinal cord injury unit at University Hospital in Boston, where I worked for two and half years. I used an amplified stethoscope and the ward clerk or other nurses alerted me if a patient was ringing for me. My ability to read lips made me good at caring for many patients on respirators. Reports were always given face-to-face. Other nurses made my phone calls and we used a "barter" system in supporting each other, as it often took more than one nurse to care for one patient.

I sought out places where members of the Deaf community gathered in Boston. Because I could read lips and speak, one Deaf person rudely told me that I was not welcome into their community. I did not let this stop me. After all, I shared their experiences and language. In 1982, I met a Deaf man at a conference whom I befriended. At his urging, I moved to Connecticut, where I found myself welcomed by both older and younger generations of Deaf people at a local social club of the Deaf.

I started working as a pediatric nurse at John Dempsey Hospital. Many parents of sick, chronically ill or disabled children held me in high esteem. While I did not consider myself disabled or ill, they saw me as proof of what their own children might be able to achieve despite their disabilities or illnesses. They would ask me what it was like growing up different and what it would mean for their child to grow up different. They wanted to know what they could do to help their children. My advice was always treat their children normally, be encouraging and supportive no matter what, and to expect them to face others who may not support their dreams.

The nursing unit in which I worked was circular, with the nurses' station in the middle. This is an ideal situation for a nurse who is Deaf. I used an amplified stethoscope, digital blood pressure machine and a master alarm with a remote receiver. I placed a receiver on IV machines or respirators to alert me via flashing lights when it rang. The receivers had lights, so I could see which room it was coming from.

When I learned about a mental health program for the Deaf at Connecticut Valley Hospital in 1983, I inquired about a position. The director hired me because I was fluent in sign language. The patients felt comfortable with me. They felt that I understood them better because I was Deaf like they were.

There, I continued to use an amplified stethoscope, digital blood pressure machines, interpreters, flashing lights and a pager. It also helped that some of the staff signed. The staff members were thrilled to have me, but the first two years were difficult because I worked with a head nurse who, perhaps, felt intimidated by me. I became a head nurse of the inpatient unit in 1985.

By 1983, I had become tired of rotating shifts, and I wanted a job with regular, 9-5 hours Monday through Friday. At the same time, I enrolled in a master of social work program. I completed it in 1986. Throughout the program, I received interpreters and note takers as accommodations.

When in 1995, the program for which I worked became completely outpatient-based, I was transferred to an outpatient setting at Capitol Region Mental Health Center in Hartford, with a team that served Deaf and hard-of hearing clients. The Center had to install fire alarms that complied with the Americans with Disabilities Act. Staff meetings with hearing clinicians were sometimes very frustrating because we had to coordinate meetings according to the availability of interpreters.

I became interested in Dialectical Behavior Therapy for individuals with borderline personality disorder and became the first Deaf person trained to use this model. I learned about the eastern mindfulness practices and cognitive behavior therapy approaches. I was given the task of translating the training manual into Deaf-friendly language. Soon, the hearing clinicians began asking me for the materials because many of their clients, who were considered severely, persistently, mentally ill, found them easy to follow and understand.

At this time, I am involved with a team from the University of Connecticut Health Center's Psychiatry department, a Deaf coworker and a hearing coworker in designing a trauma recovery group curriculum that will soon be published. I have been asked to travel to various states to provide training to staff at other mental health programs for the Deaf on dialectical behavioral therapy and trauma recovery. My trainings are usually for mental health agencies that offer Deaf services. I often use voice interpreters and communication access real-time translation at national conferences.

In 1983, while playing on a women's softball team for a local Deaf Club, I met my future husband, who was playing on the men's team. He was just starting to become exposed to the cultural view of Deafness after being raised from the pathological viewpoint. I was involved with sports, politics and social aspects within the Deaf community. My husband later played on a water polo team in the Deaf Olympics in 1985, where I had the opportunity to meet d/Deaf people from all over the world.

I realized how lucky I am to be in this country. In many other countries that still exclusively hold the pathological worldview, many d/Deaf people can't even go to college. My husband and I now have two "profoundly hearing" children who acquired sign and spoken language at an early age.

Technology for the d/Deaf has advanced greatly over the years. When I was young, there was no captioning for the televisions. Since 1993, all new televisions must have captioning built in. In the early 1970s, the telephones for the d/Deaf were big, cumbersome machines, the size of a small refrigerator, called Teletype for the Deaf. Now, TTYs are the size of a deck of cards and are fully portable. Instant messaging through the computer has become the preferred mode of communication.

In the early 1900s, hearing aids were horn-shaped devices held to the ear while individuals spoke loudly into the opening at the other end. Today, there a variety of high-tech, battery-operated, digital aids. In 1959 to 1967, I had two hearing aid packs harnessed onto me with wires attached to ear molds. I got behind-the-ear aids in 1970. I now have a behind-the-ear hearing aid embedded with a computer chip.

Cochlear implants, surgically implanted hearing aids, are a pathological way of fixing deafness. It is a subject of controversy in the Deaf community. When I was in my early 20s, I was offered the opportunity to get a cochlear implant. I declined the offer because of the invasiveness of the procedure and failure rates that are not published but known within the Deaf community. My husband was also offered a free cochlear implant and declined for the same reasons.

Flashing or vibrating alert systems allow d/Deaf people to know if the phone or doorbell is ringing or baby is crying. Before all of the technological advances available today, there were stories of strings being attached from babies' toes to the mothers' fingers. Today, there are hearing dogs specifically trained to respond to sounds and alert their owners.

As a nursing student, I had to take off my hearing aids each time I needed to use my amplified stethoscope. Now, there are blood pressure machines that do not require the use of a stethoscope. I am now experimenting with stethoscopes that record on a PDA. There are now also clear surgical masks being tested for visibility that would make it easier to read lips. I feel fortunate to have these and other technological advances available and look forward to applying them in my work.

I believe in a holistic approach to all aspects of healthcare. I have developed a strong interest in mindfulness, such as mediation, relaxation and visual imagery work. I have begun educating many d/Deaf individuals on what it means to be mindful. Many of the mindfulness materials are audiotapes or on videotapes or DVDs with no captioning. One of my goals is to make these materials accessible for the d/Deaf. I also practice complementary medicine, meaning that I use both natural and prescriptive remedies.

There are very few reviews of the literature on health beliefs among the d/Deaf. Generally speaking, the more educated and knowledgeable the d/Deaf person is, the better equipped he is to make informed health choices. The more incidental learning experiences that d/Deaf are denied, the more the person may be misinformed about various healthcare choices.

I feel that because of my life experiences transitioning from the dominant pathological worldview to the Deaf culture, my job experiences, and my hospitalizations, I can act as a cultural mediator. I have knowledge of pathological and cultural viewpoints and can communicate in all modalities (oral, signed English, American Sign Language and gestures) in order to meet the health needs d/Deaf patients.

My ability to recognize, adapt, and communicate with d/Deaf consumers with varied linguistic and intellectual abilities enables me to translate abstract health information into concrete terms, vital to help the d/Deaf consumer make educated choices. Because I have adopted values and beliefs from both the hearing and Deaf cultures, I feel that I am able to work closely with d/Deaf consumers, their families and health professionals particularly well.

Morag MacDonald, RN, MSW, is a nurse who is profoundly d/Deaf. She has practiced as a nurse for 28 years and has worked on spinal cord, pediatric and mental health units. Currently, she works as a clinical case manager at Capital Region Mental Health Center in Hartford, Connecticut. Morag expects to complete her MSN degree from St. Joseph's College in May 2006. Her goal is to become a psychiatric APRN. She can be reached at aprn2006@comcast.net.

Work*able* Wisdom

- **Think of the little engine that could.** Employers interviewing or considering a nurse with a disability should see what abilities the potential employee may have. Often, individuals with disabilities, as a result of their conditions, bring skills and talents to the nursing table that non-disabled nurses do not.

- **Highlight how your condition makes you especially valuable.** Make sure your employer, potential employers and colleagues know how your disability is advantageous in caring for patients.

- **Look at all of the possibilities in nursing.** From research or case management to school nursing, the key to finding a place or position that's a good fit for you is simply having the patience and perseverance to look until you find it. Morag used her Deafness to relate and provide quality care to d/Deaf patients and educate others on how to do the same.

◆   ◆   ◆

Zak, O. (1995). Various statistics concerning the deaf [WWW page]. URL http://www.zak.co.il/deaf-info/old/demographics.html

Deaf World Ministry. (1997). Pathological view vs. cultural view [WWW page]. URL http://www.frontpage.erie.net/dwm/article3.html

National Association of the Deaf. (2002). What is the difference between a deaf and a hard of hearing person? [WWW page]. URL http://www.nad.org/site/pp.asp?c=foINKQMBF&b=180410

de Halleux, C., & Poncelot, F. (2001). Congenital deafness. Not a disability. *The Lancet, 358*, 16-17.

ASLinfo. (1996). Deaf culture [WWW page]. URL http://www.ASLinfo.com/deafculture.cfm

Bat-Chava, Y. (2000). Diversity of deaf identity. *American annuals of the deaf, 145* (5), 420-428.

Tamaskar, P., Malia, T, Stern, C., Gorenflo, D., Meador, H., & Zazove, P. (2000). Preventive attitudes and beliefs of deaf and hard-of-hearing individuals. *Archives of family medicine, 9* (6), 518-520.

9

Oh My Aching Back! Nursing Following Injury

By Cynthia A. Weschke, RN, BSN, BC, CCM

I graduated from a diploma program at St. Luke's Hospital in St. Louis, Missouri, in 1980. I really did not want to be a nurse; I wanted to be a neurosurgeon. Alas, when seeking assistance from my high school counselor back in 1976, I was told that young ladies could be mothers, secretaries, teachers or nurses. I thought that "nurse" was the closest thing to "doctor," so I chose that. After year one, I *really* was convinced that this was not what I wanted to do.

I took a year off, searching, you might say, and finding that this was the best I could do. So I did the best I could. I made sure that I knew everything there was to know for each area in which I worked. Part of my journey has involved knowing everything possible. Research is a wonderful thing, especially when sleep evades you, as it does with chronic pain.

Mine has been a long journey, during which I have learned much and found support from some wonderful individuals online—people that I will never meet. There are a lot of things that I will share that very few have heard, even my parents.

God blessed me with the best parents anyone could ever want. You see, I am adopted, and the fact that these two people immediately fell in love with an 8-day-old infant amazes me.

No one else has ever held my head, held my hand and been there at all hours for any reason. This is truly unconditional love. They held me when I didn't even know that it was human contact I craved, supported my decisions—financially and otherwise—and guided me.

I have, in turn, sat at a bedside in ICU for hours holding a hand. I go to physician's appointments with them telephonically. It's a great system; they call me from the doctor's office on the cell phone and just lay it down so I can hear what is said.

They have supported my journey forward, even though physically I am going backwards. And they are the ones who encouraged my steps into the world of disabled nurses and employment.

Now for my story. On February 15, 1989, I arrived for work on the evening shift. As is usual on an oncology unit, we were full and almost everyone was getting "dosed." All the patients were at various stages in the administration cycle, so it promised to be a hectic evening. We did primary care with one certified nurse's aide to assist all the nurses. A fellow staff nurse asked me to help her transfer her new admit to the bedside commode.

The nurse had already admitted the patient and gave me report on the way to the room. The family assured the nurse that the patient was able to bear weight and would only require stand-by assistance. We went in to do the transfer. As we stood the patient to pivot, the patient became non-weight bearing, so we did the pivot very quickly, with me on one side and the other nurse on the other side. I had to prevent the patient from falling. In the process, I twisted awkwardly out of alignment.

I felt immediate pain and burning, and I heard popping noises coming from my lower back. I remember saying, "Well, there went my back." Still, I went on back to work. But by the time I had completed giving bedtime medications, I could not comfortably sit or stand. I notified the shift supervisor, who sent me home after completing an incident report. In order to return to work my next shift, I had to report to the employee health office.

The next day, I got ready for work and drove in. By the time I got there, I was in tears. The only position comfortable by this time was bending over a table at a 90-degree angle. The employee health nurse was immediately on the phone and arranged an appointment the next day with a physician. I went in for the appointment and saw the physician's assistant, who conducted an exam and ordered me to attend physical therapy. Unfortunately, physical therapy was a joke at that time. I truly feel that it did more harm than good.

The therapy consisted of ice, alternating heat, ultrasound, a transcutaneous electrical nerve stimulation (TENS) unit and "body traction." A harness was placed under my arms while I lay facedown on a tilt table. Then I was "hung" by my armpits, using my body for weight. At that time, my weight was around 245, so you can imagine how uncomfortable, verging on painful this was. I tolerated it for the prescribed six weeks. After that time, I was to have an "employee physical" to determine if I could return to work.

I failed the physical and was told that I would not be allowed to return to work. I was in too much pain and suffered too many muscle spasms. While there, I talked with the nurse and told her that I was uncomfortable seeing just the PA. The MD had never examined me. She made arrangements for me to see another provider. In the meantime, I saw an orthopedic surgeon on my own for a second opinion. According to him, my condition was guarded. But amazingly, his opinion changed to "there is nothing I can offer you" once he became my primary treating physician for workers' compensation.

At this point, everything becomes a little fuzzy. I retained an attorney, which where I live is the only way anything gets accomplished. First, my benefits were wrong; then, they suddenly stopped. I was told they had been "paying too much" and that benefits would resume "when sufficient time had passed to account for the pre-payment." That resulted in an emergency hearing. Someone at the hospital had filed on my papers that I was a nurse's aide, not a registered nurse. Eventually, I did get the benefits reinstated. At that point, I was assigned a case manager by the insurance company.

The case manager arrived while I was on two weeks of bed rest. She came out to the house for an initial interview. We agreed that she could follow me in therapy and visit as necessary. Attending doctor's visits was also part of the care. I started working hard at therapy. During one visit, my therapist and I discussed a two-day vacation with my family. The case manager agreed that I could go after much discussion of what activities I would and would not engage in.

The months passed, and suddenly we were going into the following spring. I had completed many weeks of conservative therapy at various locations, been CAT and MRI scanned, and been massaged to death. By this time, severe depression had set in, but I did not know what it was. I was gaining weight, the last possible thing I needed to add to the back problems. Not having anything to occupy my time, I started meeting friends after they got off work for a few drinks. The alcohol dulled the pain. This got to be a habit. I ended up in the hospital with a stomach virus, and I was told my liver enzymes were sky-high. I had to either stop this "social" drinking or die. I have not had a drink since. I don't believe I was alcohol dependent, but I might have become so.

By now, I had been treated with everything with the exception of surgery. A decompression laminectomy with a multi-level fusion and possibly Harrington rods was the remaining option. I did not see that as a valid option. The procedure scared me to death, and my weight would not allow a "reputable" surgeon to cut me or a good anesthesiologist to put me under. The procedure involved removing part of the bones in the lumbar vertebrae that protect the spinal cord, fusing the vertebrae together so there is no movement, and placing steel rods.

I decided to inquire about pain management. Initially, this was not even a consideration, mainly because no one talked to me about it. I asked my doctor many questions before agreeing to give it a try. I was to have a series of three epidural installations of steroid medications to relieve the pain. The injections themselves were a breeze. The after-effects were not. No one warned me that the medications would travel the nerves to the inflammation and that there would be severe, burning pain when the medications "landed." Those 48 hours after the injections I experienced the most severe pain I have ever had. Somehow, I made it through all three epidural installations.

I was one of the fortunate "receptive" individuals. My pain was gone. I would be able to return to work, though not work as I knew it. I could not lift more than 10 pounds, I could not bend repetitively, nor twist, squat or kneel. Think about 10 pounds. A gallon of milk weighs approximately five pounds, a sack of sugar is four pounds, and babies weigh 10 pounds by the time they are 4 months old, at minimum. What kind of work could I find?

My final hearing was in April of 1991. I was considered to be at "Maximum Medical Improvement." At that time, there were no other viable treatment options. The physician doing the rating examination rated me 50% permanently disabled, subtracting 5% for preexisting obesity. The workers' compensation judge decided that all I deserved was 20%. Part of the process is also filing for SSI or SSDI.

The SSI interview occurred over the phone, fortunately, because I was on bed rest. It happened right after I retained an attorney. The outcome decision was that since I could still talk and my thumb worked, I could dispatch cabs for a living.

I hope the vocational rehabilitation system has improved. The people I encountered had no understanding of what it's like to be homebound or on bed rest. They simply scheduled the appointment and expected me to arrive at the office. I went for my appointment and spent more than five hours there. Again, I was told that there was nothing I could retrain for that would pay me the salary I was used to. What a pickle I was in. The very programs created to assist injured workers were doing everything, it seemed, to not help at all. I became more depressed and began eating more.

Despite that, I started interviewing again. During the interviews, I did my best to ask situational questions to try and determine the lifting I would be expected to do. Eventually, I did find work as a supervisor in a nursing home. But there were so many things wrong (unsafe) that I felt like my nursing license was on the line. I actually got fired for feeding a resident. I was the only staff in the dining room with many residents. I began feeding one of the residents. I was told that since I "could not feed the residents all at once, I should not have started feeding one resident until all of the staff arrived to feed the remaining residents." I was glad to go.

Reading the want ads one day, I spotted one for a new home care company recruiting registered nurses. I sent in my resume and got an interview. At that point they had certified nurse's assistants in all the homes requiring lifting, so that was not an issue. I was called back for a second interview and was hired. I enjoyed the work, but the environment was poisonous. Looking back, it amazes me how much I have been willing to put up with in order to work. I lasted about a year before financial issues with the company became evident. Paychecks bounced and mileage checks were "lost."

I again began to look for work. I was not having any physical problems at that time, and being young, I thought the worst was over. My next position was in public health, visiting high-risk pregnant women and following them for a year post-delivery. After about three years of multiple flights of stairs in and out of apartment buildings, carrying a baby scale and a bag of supplies, I started having physical problems again. My back started to bother me, I was short of breath and the nerves in my leg were hot again. I transferred into the clinic where the environment was controlled and there were no stairs.

After five years, my manager left and recruited me to her new employer. I took a position as an obstetrical case manager for the second largest Medicaid HMO in the city of St. Louis. I loved my job. It was in an office, with no stairs, but I was sitting the better part of the day. This was hard on my back. The chairs were all wrong, and the workstations were not ergonomically designed. I know all of this now, but I had no idea then. My caseload was up to 600 at any given time.

I worked my way up the system. Then management changed. My comfort circle was gone, and I had to prove myself to new people. The manager I reported to made it clear almost immediately that I was not going out to community events or anywhere else where I would represent the company. In her words, I "did not clean up too good." That meant that she thought I was too fat and walked funny. I did eventually hear her use those exact words.

One of the things she wanted me to do was to go out to the facilities and make rounds with the concurrent reviewers. Once I explained to her that I could not walk that much, she had no interest in me as a staff person or even as a human being. I was replaced while I was out on leave of absence for carpal tunnel surgery. I returned to work to find my desk moved to the other side of the floor into a department where I knew no one.

That September (2002), I re-injured my back. At first, there was concern about a possible fractured acetabulum. But that was ruled out. The next work up was for compression fractures. By this time, ambulation was next to impossible. I was using a rolling desk chair at home and my desk chair at work to get around. One day, I had to cross the lobby to get to a meeting. I knew the chairs in the room would be too small for my girth, so I walked over, rolling my chair. My manager saw me sitting on the chair and assumed that I had rolled over in my chair. "You will walk when you are here or else you will be leaving," she demanded in front of everyone. She then asked me why I brought my chair, but before I could answer, she stated, "Oh, I know, your ass is too fat." This was in front of all the staff and some vice presidents from our parent companies. After that, I rarely saw her.

The only time I heard from her was when she needed something from me. When the company announced that it was electing not to renew the contract with the state to provide healthcare, I stopped existing to her at all. The manager told her entire staff that she would be happy to write letters of recommendations for any of her staff—except for me. I asked her four times and did not even get the courtesy of a response. Thank God, I was already in counseling. I think that if the company had stayed open, I would have been fired. I was severely depressed. (See Appendix C, Dealing with a Difficult Boss.)

We were allowed to use our time at the office to write resumes, go on interviews, network, etc. I spent a lot of time online doing research on resume writing and looking for websites specific to disabled nurses. I found a support system instead.

My goal was to locate employment. At that point, I did not care with whom or doing what for what hours. I needed an income. However, dragging through the depression was rough. Looking back, both my therapist and I firmly believe that if the company had not closed when it did, and I had not had the seven weeks of unemployment, I would have died. It would not have been at my choice, but the stress was literally killing me. It amazes me what we can withstand psychologically.

I went on an interview for a position related to workers' compensation, not knowing a thing about workers' compensation besides my personal experience. I was short of breath, in pain and very shaky in my abilities to convey what I knew and how I could be an asset to this company. I did not disclose information about my back at the interview, but I also did not hide it. If I needed to sit, I just said, "I need to stop and sit a minute."

Two weeks later, I was called with an offer and I accepted. I started work early in 2003 and ironically, I now manage the cases of injured workers. I have never felt so welcomed anywhere in my life. Even my "real" extended family is not that accepting. My manager and supervisors are wonderful. I am allowed to use my chair for transportation. I have flex hours. My coworkers are considerate of my limitations. When the pain I had from the re-injury got bad enough to see a neurosurgeon, I spoke with all of my managers.

I had an article published in *Care Management, the Journal of the Academy of Certified Case Managers* on the role of disabled nurses in bridging the nursing shortage. I took the article to work and bragged on myself. I also posted the article on a discussion group for my fellow nurses with disabilities to read. It led to discussion within my company and its parent company about how nurses can still function in nursing without necessarily engaging in direct patient care.

The article also paved the way for discussion about my own situation. I was leery that being a new employee who needs expensive medical care would be an issue. I thought I would be punished somehow. But that is far from what happened. My coworkers have covered hours for me, and my supervisors have been as accommodating as one could hope.

I have now had the first in another series of epidural steroid injections, and I'm feeling very blessed. My story is not earth shattering—it is not dramatic—but it is mine. I have fought long and hard to remain employed and to be productive. I am grateful for family and a few close friends for standing by me.

My parents are elderly, but they've stood by me in every way. Even now, my Mom does my laundry, since my washer and dryer require descending and climbing stairs. They have taken me to doctor's appointments, suffered with me, held my hand through many frightening tests and prayed for me. My counselor has been a counselor, a friend and an avid supporter. When I wrote my resume, she cried out of pride for what I had accomplished. When my article was published, she cried for joy.

It is my dream and my wish for every disabled or injured healthcare worker to have the chance to return to the workforce as a productive member of our society. Some of us will never return to work because injuries or illnesses are too severe. Others may only work for four hours a day. But I hope that through my fight, I have paved the way for others. I know that I am taking every opportunity to share our collective feelings and educate all the people I can.

Cynthia A. Weschke, RN, BSN, BC, CCM, began her career in nursing in Columbia, Missouri, at Boone Hospital Center working in cardiology, where care was provided pre-and post-operatively for cardiac bypass surgery. She returned to St. Louis after two years to pursue a BSN from Webster University. Cynthia has practiced in the areas of maternal-child, oncology and medical-surgical nursing. Currently, she works in multi-state workers' compensation, and her disabilities are accepted as a normal part of office culture. Cynthia lives in Arnold, Missouri, just south of St. Louis, and works as a telephonic nurse case manager for HealthDirect, Inc. She can be reached at cwernc@juno.com.

Work*able* Wisdom

- **Keep your head up.** If you are a nurse with a disability, know that there is no reason to watch the ground. Your condition makes you no less valuable a person or employee, even if a supervisor makes it a point to tell you otherwise.

- **Explore the world, and be assertive when looking for work.** If you are ever uncomfortable working somewhere, look for other work. It is out there.

- **Become the resident expert.** When you get a job, learn all you can about the company, its policies and rules, and the services provided. Very soon, your opinion will be sought, and you will become an indispensable part of the team.

◆　　　◆　　　◆

Weschke, C. (2003). Up front and personal. *Care management, journal of the academy of certified case managers 9* (3), 50.

Weschke, C. (2003). RNs with disabilities miss nursing. *Missouri Nurses Association, District Three Profile.*

10

Cool Nurse on Wheels: Nursing with Spina Bifida and a Wheelchair

By Marianne Haugh, RN, BSN

In April of 1983, my parents were expecting to become the parents of a healthy baby girl. However, that turned out to not be the case. I came into the world early. The doctor who was supposed to deliver me showed up at the hospital after I was born, still in his pajamas with his socks in his pocket. I was rushed from a small town hospital in Findlay, Ohio, to one in Toledo because I was born with Spina Bifida.

Once in Toledo, the rush was on to save my life. I was immediately taken into surgery, where the doctors spent an entire day working to repair the Spina Bifida as best as they could. My mother stayed behind in Findlay to recover from childbirth while my father went to be with me in Toledo. While I was in surgery fighting for my life, my parents had no idea what to expect for their new daughter.

I was born with a form of Spina Bifida called myelomeningocele. The covering of my spinal cord and the spinal nerves from L4-L5 were in a sack outside of my back, creating permanent nerve damage from the area of L4 down. Once the covering of the spinal cord and nerves were put back into my body, I developed a condition called hydrocephalus. The cerebrospinal fluid had nowhere to go, so it built up in my brain. Thus, the second surgery I had was to insert a shunt—a tube extending from my brain into my abdomen used to drain the fluid from my brain. This lessened my chances of having brain damage from the fluid build-up. So began my life, full of multiple hospitalizations and surgeries.

Growing up, my older brother was my protector. Josh and I are seven years apart, but we've grown closer over time. He helped me with my schoolwork when I needed to catch up after a hospitalization. He never treated me as his "sick" little sister. I was just his kid sister, who happened to need a little help walking.

Even though my brother and I were—and still are—two very different people, our parents always enforced the same rules for both of us. If my brother got in trouble for something, and I did the same thing, I got in trouble for it as well. My family raised me with a "can do" attitude, and I was never treated any differently than the other kids in my family. We never focused on what I could not do: I was raised to always focus on what I could do. Even if I could not run, I could still do lots of other things that other kids could do.

This attitude shaped who I am now. I always figure out how I can best do what I want to do. I tend to be defiant and figure out how to do something that I am told either not to do or that I cannot do. Sometimes that defiance got me into trouble at home. But at the same time, it has helped me be persistent and reach for my goals in life, no matter what they are.

Becoming a nurse was the ultimate goal for me; and from day one, I was not going to let anyone or anything stand in my way. I have wanted to be a nurse ever since I can remember. It's my calling. It's what I was born to do. As strange as it may sound, a part of me always felt like I belonged in the hospital, even as a patient. I never enjoyed the pain I endured during my many hospital stays, but I still felt that I belonged there. I paid close attention to every detail of the care that the nurses gave me, and I always asked a ton of questions. Sometimes the nurses were nice enough to explain what they were doing and why, but sometimes they wouldn't really talk to me. My mom and I nicknamed a nurse I had often, "Sergeant Carol," because she was just like a drill sergeant. When she was my nurse, I wasn't allowed to act like a little kid. She was all business. Luckily, not all of my nurses were like her.

During all the times I've been a patient, I have never slept in a hospital except for when I've been medicated. I've always been afraid that someone would do something to me while I slept, such as give me the wrong drug or perform some painful procedure without first warning me. I didn't want to miss a thing. Sleeping was something to do once I got home.

As I progressed through high school, I began to consider what college to attend. During a spring break visit to my brother's house, I had an interview with a nursing school. The morning of the interview, the nursing school called the person in disability services that had set up my interview and told her not to send me over because they had heard that I used a wheelchair. I was devastated. This was only the beginning of my troubles.

My mom got a new job the summer before my senior year in high school, so I relocated to South Carolina for my last year. During that year, I e-mailed several nursing schools in and around the state to find out whether they would be open to admitting a student who was in a wheelchair into their nursing programs. All of the responses were negative. Some schools even offered me free counseling to change my major. I had the test scores and grades to get into these schools, but they concluded that I was choosing the wrong major. Most of the college representatives I spoke with said that I would be a great social work or education major but not a nursing major. One told me that a clinical setting was no place for a wheelchair. You can't tell me that there are no wheelchairs in hospitals!

The only school I applied to was Wright State University. I decided not to disclose my Spina Bifida until necessary. I was accepted with nursing as my major. The first time I met with my academic advisor to choose classes, no negative thoughts were expressed about my intended major. In fact, we discussed which track of nursing to take. I decided on the track that would allow me to complete the program in just three years. My academic advisor supported my choice at that point. I felt so relieved.

Next, I had to apply to the college of nursing itself. Again, I faced the issue of disclosure. I decided to disclose my Spina Bifida in the essay that I was required to submit as part of the college of nursing application. The topic was why I wanted to go into nursing, so I explained my numerous surgeries and hospitalizations. I was elated when I got the letter of admittance.

During my first quarter of nursing school, one of my professors suggested that I meet the assistant dean of the nursing college. I was very nervous about what she would say to me. I had made it this far, but I was still a little afraid that she was going to tell me that nursing wasn't for me. Instead, she vowed to help me in any way that she could. We decided that since this was going to be a new experience for both of us, we would take it quarter by quarter, meeting prior to the start of each clinical to assess any potential obstacles. We knew that we were going to have to pick apart each clinical and assess whether or not I absolutely had to perform every skill. If it was not an essential function for nursing, then we discussed delegating the task to someone else. If I knew there was a lift or transfer that I could not perform, I asked a classmate to do it for me, promising to lend my help when he or she needed it.

While Wright State was willing to work with me in a clinical setting right from the start, the hospital I was placed in for my first clinical was not so accommodating. My first clinical instructor met with someone from the hospital and was told that I would have to have a nurse with me at all times. Otherwise, the hospital would not have me there as a student. I'm not sure what they thought I was going to do if I was by myself, but they were obviously afraid of something. I was, therefore, assigned a new nurse, Mary, who had recently graduated from Wright State.

She never helped me with any of the skills I needed to perform, but she did explain things to me when my instructor was not available. Other students also came to Mary with questions. Still, the hospital was strict about my presence there. My friend, Becky, was even asked to "watch" me once when Mary was down the hall. I think the hospital expected me to need more physical help than I actually did. Finally after two quarters, the hospital agreed that I didn't need Mary constantly at my side.

During my geriatric clinical, I was also assigned nurses to help me with any lifting or transferring. But after a few weeks of not really needing much help, that was discontinued as well. From that point on, my clinical instructors and I just decided that I would ask my fellow nursing students for any help I might need. The arrangement worked well.

When the time came to choose what area I wanted to be in for my final practicum, I chose the newborn intensive care unit. I thought it would be great to work with the tiny babies, and it might be easier on me physically, since I wouldn't have any patients bigger than 10 pounds. Most of these babies only weighed one to three pounds. Some were on ventilators because they were too young to breathe on their own. After being in the NICU for my final three months of nursing school, I decided that I no longer wanted to do NICU nursing. I felt uncomfortable working with the babies on ventilators. With that decision, the job search began.

I wanted to stay close to my friends and family after graduation, so I decided to look for jobs around Dayton, where most of my friends were staying. I scheduled a few interviews in the area. My first one was for a pediatric psych position. It was there that I got my first taste of what was to come.

I had decided not to disclose any information about the Spina Bifida prior to the interview. As the interview progressed, I thought it was going very well. I really started to think that I might get the job. I had another interview for a labor and delivery position lined up a few days later. It was after that interview that I was finally called back about the first job. I was in my car when my cell phone rang. It was the lady from human resources. She told me that the nurse manager of the psych unit, whom I had never met in person, decided that her unit was not a good fit for me because I would not be able to handle "take downs," if they came up. This nurse manager had never met or spoken to me, so how she knew my abilities (or lack of abilities), I don't know. I called my mom crying. Little did I know there was more to come.

I graduated from Wright State in November 2004. Up until the summer of 2005, I was interviewing constantly. I interviewed at numerous hospitals and even worked with some nurse recruiters, but I got turned down for every job. I disclosed my Spina Bifida before some interviews; for others, I did not say anything until I went into the interview room.

The excuses for me not getting the jobs ranged from, "We want someone with more experience," even though they advertised the job for new graduates, to "You can't possibly do nursing with a wheelchair." It was amazing how many nurse recruiters I spoke with never returned my calls after I disclosed my Spina Bifida. One hospital in South Carolina even told me that they were in a hiring freeze after I had just completed two interviews there. I spent most of the spring in Indianapolis with a friend interviewing for positions from labor and delivery to pediatric hematology/oncology. The feedback I got was that I was good at interviewing but not good enough to be a nurse.

Finally, in summer 2005, I went back to Wright State and met with people from the disability services office and the assistant dean of the nursing college. We discussed interview techniques and tried to figure out why I didn't have a job yet. Everyone else that I graduated with had one. I had another set of interviews coming up soon in Chicago, so we tried to prepare for those as well. We also agreed to team up to help the next person with a wheelchair who decides to go through the nursing program.

In June 2005, I had filled out an online application for the Rehabilitation Institute of Chicago. The gentleman from human resources called me right back. He used to work at the hospital where I had done my clinicals. For some reason, I felt comfortable disclosing my Spina Bifida over the phone. I told him that I was interested in spinal cord injuries and rehabilitation because of my history with Spina Bifida. He immediately asked me to come to Chicago and interview. I flew out to interview for this position and one at another hospital.

The interview at the other hospital did not go very well, but I spent all day at RIC interviewing for two different positions. One was for a position on the pediatric floor. I was very excited when I walked out of that interview because I knew it had gone well. I was to fly back to Ohio the next day. I wasn't even out of the airport parking garage when I got a phone call requesting a second interview with the pediatric floor. I flew back to Chicago, where I shadowed on the unit for a day and was offered a job as a staff nurse a few weeks later. I gladly accepted.

I now work at RIC as a full-time registered nurse, and it has been a great experience. I use my wheelchair for long distances, such as in the hallway, but I do walk in my patients' rooms. The only accommodation that RIC has really had to make for me is getting me latex-free sterile gloves to use for suctioning. Since I have a latex allergy, I try my best to stay away from latex as much as possible. But latex gloves are still in use there, so I carry around a box of clean latex-free gloves with me everywhere. For the most part, my patients have been very accepting of a nurse with a wheelchair. A lot of my younger patients think it is cool that their nurse has a wheelchair just like them.

I graduated in November 2004. It was the proudest day of my life. As I walked across the stage, I had tears in my eyes because I knew that I had achieved my dream. Nursing school was rough, and I learned to really rely on my friends and family for support. I made a lot of great friends during those years, and I could not have made it without their support and encouragement. The biggest lesson that I have learned from this entire experience is to never let go of a dream. No matter what the dream is, if you focus on it and keep reaching for it, then you can achieve it.

Marianne Haugh, RN, BSN, was born in Ohio and graduated from the BSN program at Wright State University. She is currently a staff nurse on the pediatric unit of the Rehabilitation Institute of Chicago. She can be reached at mkhaugh@hotmail.com.

Work*able* Wisdom

- **Be persistent.** Whether it's finding a nursing school willing to support you or an employer who will give you a chance to prove your abilities, the key is to keep looking. Don't let one or two or three failed interviews or college applications keep you from what you know you can do.

- **Communicate with your superiors.** In school, your professors and administrators can be great advocates. Get them on your side early on by showing them that you are as able to have a nursing career as any other student there.

- **Keep an open mind when searching for a job.** If you narrow your job search by location or by the kind of unit where you would like to work, you also narrow your chances of finding a job. The unfortunate reality is that many hospital administrators and human resource personnel will discriminate against a nurse with disabilities.

11

Disability as a Gift: Nursing with AIDS

By G.C.S., LPN

My career into nursing happened quite by accident. I was born and raised in rural North Carolina. There were not a lot of opportunities for me in school, since my family did not focus on education. My father quit school in the sixth grade, and my mother quit in the eighth grade. They both came from uneducated families where the focus was work and survival. I was raised under a strict religious ethic that focused primarily on serving God and the church. Our lives were only focused on the church. My parents' religion is Pentecostal Holiness, a very strict, cult-like religion. You were to never question life or the path you were on. I also was indoctrinated on the premise that you are to be obedient to your parents, community and job. Change was not a good thing. For me, there was no change.

After finishing high school and working 11 years in a local burger barn, I decided to make a break for it. I left not just my family, job and partner at the time, but the many years of stagnation. I moved to Florida. I got up one morning, drove straight through to the city of Lakeland, found a small apartment, drove back to North Carolina the next day, packed up and moved. I had no idea what I was doing, but I knew it had to be done. I had no friends, family or anyone to support me in Florida, but I moved anyway.

The first year was hard. My parents didn't like the fact that I had moved away. But I survived. I continued working in the burger business and moved up the corporate ladder. When the business folded, I found myself without a job and any education to fall back on. In 1990, I started attending a local junior college. Since my grades and educational background were not so good, I had to start at the very bottom. I had no confidence or the self-discipline to study. I didn't know where to start. A person I befriended guided me and slowly helped me gain the confidence to pursue an education. And so I did. Through all the ups and downs, I survived.

I finally realized that no matter what you have as possessions, an education is the most priceless. I'm thankful and grateful for everyone who has helped me get this far with my education. I'm currently a licensed practical nurse and am finishing my studies to become a registered nurse. I've been an LPN since 1994 and have enjoyed every day, though some have been more challenging than others. I work at a large hospital in Florida.

As a male nurse with the human immunodeficiency virus, I face more challenges than the average nurse. As a male nurse, some people expect you to perform more physical work. Most female nurses call upon you to lift patients or to handle hostile situations with patients or family members. But being a male nurse also has its advantages. I personally believe most male nurses are less afraid to ask for higher pay or raises, and they speak up more about work environment situations. Most of the male nurses I've worked with come from a business or military background. They are not afraid to ask, question or seek out answers through the chain of command. Female nurses are learning this from us. Being aggressive in your job does not mean you have to be unprofessional.

As for being HIV+, I face many daily obstacles. One obstacle is taking care of patients who can easily make me sick. I always use and follow universal precautions, which protect both my patients and me. Second, I know myself, my body and my health. I never push myself harder than I know I should. I work only 40 hours per week, eat right, sleep and take my medications. I follow my doctor's instructions and get regular check ups. If I need rest, I rest. If I'm sick, I stay home. That's why most employers have sick days and offer family and medical leave. I don't abuse my sick time, but I do use it when I need it. Third, I stay informed on new treatments. What works today may not work tomorrow.

I keep my nurse manager and employee health department informed of any needs I may have. I have asked for and been granted accommodation in the past. I asked not to work on a specific unit, which I found to be more physically demanding than others. I never hesitate to ask for anything to protect my patients or me. (See Appendix A, Sample Accommodation Request Letter.)

I know I have more than the average nurse to contribute to the profession. I do it every day. As a nurse with HIV and one who has gone through the maze and humiliation of the Welfare system, I have much wisdom to offer my patients and fellow nurses. I have lost friends, family and coworkers to HIV. No, I didn't lose them to untimely death. I lost them due to the ignorance and fear of HIV/ AIDS. There is a stigma of living with HIV that is portrayed through the media.

The stigma is that a person with HIV is a person who uses IV drugs, has unsafe sex with multiple partners and lives life on the edge. While this may be true for a small few, we cannot all be placed in the same box. Some with HIV, like myself, acquired it through love and trust—a big price for a meaningful relationship.

When I was diagnosed, my T-cell count was 30 (normal should be above 600). I was working as a licensed practical nurse and enrolled in an RN program. When told I only had six months to live, I decided to go on a leave of absence from my job to travel and rest. I started taking the HIV meds, put school on hold, cashed in all my life insurance policies and started my journey as a person with AIDS. I went on Social Security Disability, SSI and Medicare/Medipass. I felt like a leper. I had few outlets for social stimulation except the HIV/AIDS support group. I lived on $1,000 per month. This had to cover rent, utilities, a car payment and co-pays for medications and doctor's visits. I had little left for food or other needs.

For almost two years, I was on Welfare. The Community AIDS Network helped with groceries and my personal needs. I lost weight, had many reactions to medications and stayed in bed most of the time.

Finally, I realized that I was not going to die. I decided to go back to work, though this was no easy task. A nurse diagnosed with AIDS is not someone an institution wants on its payroll, despite the fact that there are no known cases where the virus has been transmitted from nurse to patient. I don't do invasive procedures that could put my patients or me at risk. After much persuasion and networking, I came off leave of absence and started working part-time. A year passed, and I was doing fine. My T-cell count was slowly climbing, so I started to work full-time.

In 2003, I found an online, self-paced RN program that works well for me. I will be finished with the program by the end of this year. The journey to become an RN will have taken me 15 years.

I have taken care of patients who were newly diagnosed with HIV and felt their shock and disbelief. When a doctor or nurse practitioner gives such news to a patient, the professional can only think and explain it in technical medical terms. Healthcare professionals cannot feel what it is like to be told you have a chronic disease—one that cannot be cured with today's advanced medical care.

As the doctor leaves the room and the patient is left alone to ponder what happens now, I can step in. I remember when I was told the devastating news, "You have HIV." Back then, I had no one to turn to.

Now, I have the greatest gift of all to share. I've been there, experienced it, have it, and know the different treatment plans, and I'm a survivor. I have referred many of my patients to the appropriate agencies to help them obtain education about HIV, care and support groups. I listen to the disbelief of, "How did this happen?" When I disclose my status, I always hear the same thing, "You don't look sick." My response is, "I didn't know I was supposed to look sick." Then we both laugh. Again, I hear the stigma. People with HIV are supposed to look sick. What better education could there be than seeing and talking to a real person who has experienced everything a patient is about to?

When you live with a chronic disease day in and day out, you become familiar with what is changing in your body and in your life. You can share and educate your patients and coworkers just by showing up for work and setting a positive example. Over time, people learn to see you in a different light—not as a person with a chronic illness, but a person who takes life and runs with it into their dreams. I am that person. I go to work every day; and by going to work, I'm contributing to the profession of nursing and to the reputation of all people with disabilities. I'm a daily example that if you decide to take charge of your life and health, you can do anything, no matter what type of disability you may have.

To other nurses or students with HIV, I suggest that you don't disclose your status when enrolling in school or searching for a job. You will have to have a complete physical before entering nursing school or prior to employment. Your physical condition and health is all that needs to be documented by you and your doctor. As for employment, there is no need to disclose if you are going to practice in an environment that does not include any invasive procedures. Before embarking on any career in healthcare, check the Centers for Disease Control and Prevention guidelines for persons with HIV working in healthcare. Every hospital should have policies and procedures in place for workers who are exposed to or have HIV. If you follow the CDC guidelines, you won't put anyone at risk.

As I continue my career in nursing and my journey with HIV, I know I will have only more to offer my patients and coworkers. I now have diabetes, hypertension and lipoatrophy—all caused by HIV. Each is a disability in its own right. My example of living life to the fullest and not giving up no matter how difficult or challenging it may become will only help erase the stigma associated with disability. To have a disability, I believe, is to receive a gift.

When you are given this gift, you can either choose to keep it wrapped up or open it up and learn to use it to help others. By choosing to open your gift and share your experiences with others, you begin the process of education, ending discrimination against persons with disabilities and becoming a role model. It's easy to sit on the sidelines, do nothing and watch the world go by. It's hard to get on the court with a disability and play. But with the right tools, education and support, everyone with a disability can play.

When I question, "Why am I here God?" I now know the answer. I am here to share my positive gift with everyone.

* Portions of this chapter appear in Minority Nurse *(Spring 2006).*

G.C.S., LPN, was born in North Carolina and started his career in nursing as an LPN later in life. He lives in Florida. His name, work place, or other personally identifying information have been withheld due to his fear of consequences. He is an activist for ending HIV/AIDS discrimination and a supporter of gay, lesbian, bisexual and transgender causes. He received the 2005 Nurse of the Year Award from the neuroscience unit at his place of employment.

Work*able* Wisdom

- **Work to prove the stigma wrong.** Individuals with chronic diseases like HIV will most likely face stigma in the workplace and in life in general. By making others see that you are nothing like the stereotypes, you are creating a better working environment for yourself and making it easier for those like you who will follow.

- **Don't let grim medical predictions slow you.** Doctors are sometimes wrong. If you let a grim medical prediction take over your life, you are wasting precious time that could be spent furthering your education or helping others. When it comes to dealing with chronic illness, the best approach is preparing for both the worst and the best.

- **Consider keeping your disability to yourself in certain instances.** If your condition doesn't have the potential of putting patients at risk and you need no accommodations to perform your job, there may be no reason to disclose to an employer.

12

Quitting Is Not an Option: Nursing with Dystonia

By Rebecca Serdans, RN, BSN, MSN, ANP

It all began with a stiff neck. A movement disorder specialist first diagnosed dystonia in 1995, although looking back, I recall my father making remarks about abnormal movements, tremors and twitches when I was 18 or 19 years old. I've dealt with dystonia for practically half my life, but it did not get correctly diagnosed until I was 28 years old. It seems like I've had this forever. I can no longer remember what is normal and what is not.

Dystonia is a neurological disorder classified as a movement disorder. It falls within the Parkinson's disease tremor continuum. More than 350,000 people in North America have the disease, but it often goes undiagnosed because it resembles other movement disorders. Plus, many healthcare specialists are unfamiliar with the disorder. It's not unusual for patients to go without a diagnosis for an extended period of time. Little did I know at the time how my life would change when I was diagnosed.

I am of European descent. My entire family emigrated from Latvia, a Baltic State, to both Germany and the United States during the 1940s, when everyone was trying to outrun both the Germans and Russians. I was born in Germany and lived there for several years; thus, I am fluent in several languages. By age 6, I came to the U.S., although I have spent a good deal of time in Europe since then.

I am the oldest of three girls and the only one with dystonia. My two siblings are fit and healthy, which at times I envy. I sometimes struggle with the "Why me?" question. Not knowing why can be torturous to the mind and the body.

Upon the urging of my father, I entered nursing school and graduated from the University of Rochester with a BSN and pre-med studies. After spending six months working on a cardiac telemetry unit, I entered critical care nursing. I like the analytical and technical aspect of critical care nursing.

Symptoms of dystonia developed slowly over time. I began experiencing abnormal movements of the neck, facial spasms, blepharospasms and walking difficulties, along with dysphonia, known as dystonia of the vocal cords, which gave me a light breathy voice quality.

I diagnosed myself by opening a textbook on neurology and finding a picture of a woman with similar symptoms. Despite visits to several physicians, dystonia was not officially diagnosed until I sought help from Mount Sinai's Movement Disorder Center in New York City. The disorder was suspected in 1994 at the University of Rochester Medical Center, but the complexity of my symptoms baffled the physicians.

Initially, I shuttled between Rochester and New York City for treatment, but I eventually moved to the city, arriving at NewYork-Presbyterian. Up to this point, I had been working full-time within critical care, sometimes wearing cervical collars and splints for 12 hours.

I began treatment with botulinum toxin (Botox A) in 1995. I also entered several clinical trials using other drugs, all of which failed. Today, I carry the diagnosis of having primary dystonia, dysphonia and torticollis (cervical)—three distinct forms of dystonia.

I received botulinum toxin A and B at the Neurological Institute affiliated with Columbia Medical Center. Botulinum toxins temporarily block nerve impulses that induce constant muscle contractions that cause the signs of dystonia. The toxin is injected every three months in the most active muscles, so treatment is chronic and life-long, as long as one doesn't develop antibodies to the toxin. A cure does not exist. The mechanics of the disease are not yet completely understood, although a gene has been identified in childhood-onset dystonia. I underwent genetic testing, which proved to be useless, since the gene occurs in only about 5% of those diagnosed with generalized dystonia.

Working as a nurse while having a movement disorder is difficult. I don't think most people realize how difficult it is to work with a "visible" disease. One can hide diabetes and a glucometer, but one can't hide tremors, pain, abnormal twitching and posturing. With dystonia, one learns to use "sensory tricks"—body postures that allow one to hide the abnormal movements—to hide the disease, but this works only for so long. Actor Michael J. Fox was able to do so for seven years. The same applies to me. There is not a day when I do not think about when I no longer will be able to practice critical care nursing.

Many of my colleagues in the ICU do not comprehend dystonia or the amount of effort it takes to hide the abnormal movements and to compensate for those movements. I no longer work in the post anesthesia care unit because pushing beds is immensely difficult. I end up steering beds with patients into walls and making dents along the hallways.

Walking can be tiresome, as the task of "gait" involves spatial orientation and coordination. I walk into walls, cut into corners, and can't always open or crush medications. It's difficult to focus on tasks as brain signals are firing to muscles, inducing the abnormal movements. Using two hands at the same time is difficult. Motor coordination is no longer smooth and refined. Despite these few examples, I rarely ask for help from my colleagues. I have developed a way of nursing that motivates my patients to help me, which only helps them in their own recovery. I haven't asked for any work accommodations.

Patients constantly ask what is wrong with me. At times, I simply say, "a stiff neck." If they question me a bit more, I explain dystonia to them. You would think that I would be embarrassed to work with patients, but I am not because they see a quality of nursing not given to them by others. This is not to say that my colleagues provide poor care—they don't—but they can't connect with patients on an emotional level—one that hits the soul. You cannot learn this unless you have been a patient as well as a nurse.

Personally I am more embarrassed by being out on the street, because a social stigma exists when one looks different. It is pervasive in today's society. Some people are so afraid of others with a disability that they make every attempt to avoid you. They react to you as if you have the plague. I feel safer within the hospital setting, as I have educated everyone about dystonia. Still, they don't live with it on a daily basis, so there is much they don't know. Knowing symptoms is quite different from living with symptoms. But educating others transforms plague-like reactions to cooperative pleasantness.

I would not be able to continue working as a critical care nurse if I did not have the support of everyone at work—nursing, medical staff and others. There are high rates of depression, disability, unemployment, isolation and loss associated with dystonia. The fact that my colleagues are not embarrassed by me and are able to see beyond the movements helps considerably. It means a lot to me as I worked at an Upper East Side hospital for six months, where I was ridiculed and laughed at by the nursing staff.

I still carry my load of patients in the critical care units. I never take a break, although I do lie down for an hour before the start of the shift. Dystonia eases when you are in the horizontal position—it's the vertical position that brings on problems. No one knows the physics behind this phenomenon. I also ask for help on a more frequent basis now, since my dystonia has become highly resistant to treatment. They also know how dedicated I am to helping others who are in worse shape than me. I don't see myself as a bad case, but I know that my dystonia has progressed over the years and will most likely take me away from nursing in the future. I have begun breaking up my shifts, no longer working six-12-hour shifts in a row; instead, I work two or three with a rest day in between.

Being both a patient and a caregiver—essentially being on two sides of the coin—has brought along other job opportunities: writing books that describe my daily experiences with dystonia and working as a patient advocate and consultant for pharmaceutical companies. Being a nurse with a disease such as mine has opened up doors that have diminished the impact of the loss of previous goals and dreams. I have also obtained a master's in nursing.

As a nurse and patient, I realized that multidisciplinary care was needed for those of us with dystonia. I would sit for hours waiting for my physician and the toxin—sort of routine, like filling your gas tank. Because the entire appointment focused on toxin dosages, I would rarely get an answer to a question or simply be listened to as a patient. I got looked upon as the "nurse" or the icon in the dystonia world. But at times I simply felt like screaming that I hate this disease. Rarely did anyone ask how I was doing on an emotional and social level.

Eventually, I realized that if this was happening to me, it was happening to others. Working as a speaker for Athena Diagnostics, I met others across the country and collected information about the type of care being provided. Once my counterparts learned that I was a nurse with dystonia, out came the horror stories, which only confirmed my own. I knew that optimal dystonia care had never been identified or implemented.

That's how I came up with Care for Dystonia (www.care4dystonia.org), a nonprofit organization focused on setting the pace in areas of public awareness, patient education and collaboration.

Over time, one learns that quitting is not an option, and whining is annoying. Life goes on, even with dystonia. It does so with any disability. That's the most important advice I can give others with a disability. Employers need to learn to be attuned to their staff or employees. They should learn about each and every individual. I ask:

Is it too much to comprehend
Or ask for
Recognition of disease,
Chronic disease.

Open your eyes
And see.

Don't become blind to the needs of others.
Look beyond us,
Beyond anyone.

Never say good-bye to dreams.
They keep you going
During tough times.
Hold on to them,
And never let them go.
Keep a memory of them.
Bank upon them during times of need.

Rebecca Serdans, RN, BSN, MSN, ANP, is a specialist in critical care. She obtained her BSN from the University of Rochester. She also completed pre-med studies and wished to pursue a career in medicine prior to the diagnosis of dystonia, a movement disorder. She lives in New York and works as a per diem nurse within New York-Presbyterian's critical care division. She completed her master's in nursing in 2006 and works as an adult nurse practitioner in a cardiologist's office. Rebecca serves on medical advisory boards and dystonia nonprofit groups. She created a resource for patients called Care for Dystonia (www.care4dystonia.org) and has published three books. She was also featured on NBC's Dateline *program and other media venues. She is currently receiving treatment at the Weill-Cornell Medical Center's Surgical Movement Disorder Division after the implantation of a Deep Brain Stimulation system. Photos of the journey can be viewed at www. parasphotography.com/beka.html. She can be reached at Infoc4d@aol.com.*

Work*able* Wisdom

- **Find others like yourself.** It may seem like you are the only nurse with your condition—even other people with your condition in some cases. But go to conferences where they are likely to be or create a place on the Internet that will draw them in. There is strength—and comfort—in numbers.

- **Turn your condition into opportunities.** You can be just another person with a disability, or you can be an advocate for yourself and others with your disability. Use your expertise in the health profession to fight against stigma and poor care. Figure out what you are more qualified to do for having a disability. Can you write a book? Become a consultant? Such activities will only make you a more valuable member of your company.

- **Get on with it.** No matter the disability, there is life after disability. The longer you dwell on the things you can no longer do, the longer it will take you to find all the new things you can do.

◆   ◆   ◆

Serdans, B. (2001). *I'm moving on...are U?*. Philadelphia, PA: Xlibris Corporation.

13

Future Planning

By Donna Carol Maheady, ARNP, EdD

Let's face it. Most nurses won't work as staff nurses on medical-surgical floors for 40 years. Planning for the future should begin today. Everyone needs to explore all of the "What if?" questions about themself, their family, career and finances in order to formulate a plan of action should disability strike. Imagine that you become disabled from an accident, stroke or illness. After rehabilitation, you long to return to nursing—to the work you love. Questions may surface, such as, Will my position be there? Will accommodations be made for me if necessary?

From the experiences of the nurses included in this book, the answer is sometimes "yes" and sometimes "no." The opportunity to work as a nurse in your previous position may not be available, no matter how much experience or commitment you have.

Often, nurses are so busy caring for others that they forget about caring for themselves. Nurses should consider doing a yearly inventory or career checkup based on age, personal and family health status, finances and professional and healthcare industry trends. As a way to remember, this annual checkup might be scheduled at the start of a new year or on a birthday or anniversary. Notes could be kept in a journal. Answers to the following questions will help to formulate a personal/professional care plan:

- What if I become disabled?

- What if I'm in an accident?

- What if I hurt my back at work?

- What if a patient hits me?

- What if my disability exacerbates or is disclosed?

- What if I get sick?

- What if my parent, spouse or child gets sick?

In addition to a yearly professional checkup, nurses need to stay as healthy as possible, take care of themselves and continue to learn new skills throughout their careers. The following suggestions are similar to what nurses teach their patients every day:

- Get regular medical checkups.

- Eat healthy, exercise, laugh, play and give thanks.

- Don't drink in excess or smoke.

- Recognize when you may be burned out. These times should serve as a wake-up call to first take care of yourself so you can be of service to others.

- Reduce stress. Try yoga or a dance class. Learn a new craft or hobby, such as knitting or scrapbook making. Take a cooking class.

- Recognize your limitations. Be honest with yourself and others. Say "no" when appropriate.

- Ask yourself the tough questions: Can I perform the essential skills of the job with or without accommodations? Conduct an inventory of your strengths and weaknesses. Compare this list with the essential skills or technical standards of the nursing position you have or are considering.

- Be prepared to answer questions, such as, "How will you perform CPR? How will you lift, transfer and ambulate a patient? How will you hear a patient's call bell or the telephone?" Identify any areas of possible concern.

- Address any issues head on, with patient safety foremost in mind. Address potential concerns your employers may have by demonstrating or describing how you would meet technical standards with or without reasonable accommodations.

- Consider whether to disclose carefully. Your need to disclose your disability to your employer is proportional to your need for accommodations. It's like wearing glasses or contacts: If your vision aid sufficiently corrects your vision, then you don't need to talk about it with your employer. If you can fulfill your duties with your aids, don't make a big deal of it. If you will need to use a wheelchair, scooter, or sign language interpreter, consider informing a potential employer early in the application process.

- Be upfront and honest if you need your employer to make accommodations. But also be prepared to answer questions and deal proactively with ignorant comments or biased behavior.

- Do your homework. It is your legal responsibility to do the research and know what accommodations to ask for. Your employer isn't responsible for knowing what you need.

- Seek assistance from attorneys, advocacy organizations, union officers and other nurses with disabilities if you need to make a case for being allowed to continue practicing as a nurse.

- Study the laws that offer protection to employees with disabilities, such as the American with Disabilities Act of 1990 and the Family and Medical Leave Act of 1993.

- Familiarize yourself with the regulations and services provided by the Bureau of Workers' Compensation and your state's vocational rehabilitation agency. If you become a recipient of services from workers' compensation or vocational rehabilitation, learn all you can about the agency and services offered. There may be an employment opportunity for you within the system designed to help you.

- Visit the website of your state's nursing board. Review your state's Nurse Practice Act. Research whether or not your state has practice restrictions or a limited license for nurses with disabilities.

- Study your hospital's or employer's policies for employees. What provisions are made for nurses to return to work on light-duty assignment? Sick leave?

- Volunteer to work on a committee to develop strategies for accommodating nurses who need temporary or permanent accommodations. Work as a camp nurse for children or adults with chronic illness or disabilities. Robin Mazzuca, RN, MPH, has multiple sclerosis. She and her service dog, Georgia, volunteer at nursing homes, schools and rehabilitation facilities. Consider going with a medical mission team to another country. Volunteer to be the nurse at your local *Walk for the Cure*. Teach a class for newly diagnosed people with your disability or lead a support group. These opportunities can later turn into a new employment opportunity.

- Be a change agent. Examine the mission and value statements of your place of employment. Is dedication to employees a value? Is health promotion, safe working conditions, support, respect, loyalty, diversity, flexibility and equal opportunity included? If not, work to make changes.

- Network. Professional contacts are vital in planning for the future. When you attend meetings, conferences or continuing education programs, sit with new people and introduce yourself. Remember names. Collect business cards, names, numbers and e-mail addresses. Follow up with new contacts, and stay in touch. Friendships and successful ventures can be built by sharing ideas, resources and leads. If you become a good networker, you also become a good listener, conversationalist and resource for others—even if you're the one looking for the leads.

- Join professional organizations. Join your state's nursing association or organizations related to your disability. Attend meetings and serve on committees. Run for office. The experience and the networking opportunities will benefit you in the future.

- Learn new skills. Stay current with computer skills and the latest technology. If an in-service is offered about new equipment, try to attend. Study a foreign language or take a sign language or lip reading course.

- Continue your education. Consider working on your AD, BSN, MS or doctoral degree. Take it slow if you need to. Obtain and maintain certifications in your specialty area.

- Diversify, diversify, diversify. Whenever possible, go back to school for an advanced degree, volunteer to be a school nurse on your day off, work as a camp nurse for a week or a summer, sign up with an agency and do an occasional home visit or private duty case. Be open to other areas of nursing. While following a patient to cardiac rehab, did you get excited about the possibilities of working there?

- Be flexible. Cast a wide net when considering different opportunities. The options are endless. Consider case management, telephone triage, pharmaceutical sales, research, medical coding, medical transcription, legal nurse consulting, parish nursing, teaching, informatics, quality assurance, writing for healthcare-related publications, and school or camp nursing.

- Take care of your finances. Consider disability insurance and invest wisely (payroll deductions, IRAs). Save for that rainy day. Invest in mortgage and credit unemployment insurance, and set money aside in liquid assets—preferably at least six month's worth of income. This way, you have the cash to survive an interruption in income, and the unemployment insurance will ensure that your home and credit cards are protected during this time.

• Read and listen. Find out about new career opportunities in nursing. Attend Donna Cardillo's Career Alternatives for Nurses™ seminar or purchase a DVD, audiocassette or videotape of the presentation. After her presentation, you'll feel good and positive about yourself and your profession and be armed with information, resources and motivation to move forward in your career.

• Consider career coaching. A life or career coach may help you achieve your goals.

• Write. After a long career in nursing, Connie Stallone Adleman, RN, had a stroke. She attributes her remarkable recovery to writing. She writes continuing education programs for nurses and is writing a book about her experiences following her stroke. Following a back injury, Trenee' Carlson Zweigle, RN, wrote *Psych Ward*, a book about her experiences working in mental health settings. Patricia Holloran, RN, wrote *Walking Like a Duck* based on her personal journey from addiction to recovery. Following a work-related spinal injury, Anne Hudson, RN, and William Charney wrote *Back Injury Among Healthcare Workers*.

• Keep a journal. Journal writing is helpful to many people. Through guided questions, Ritter (2006) developed a workbook that helps to develop a self-care plan for people suffering from the loss of physical capacity. The exercises help people see how they still have strengths and abilities and can move beyond being disabled. It encourages readers not to wallow on what has been lost.

• Become your own publicist. Stories about nurses with disabilities are important. Contact your local newspaper, radio or television station. Ask them to consider doing an interview with you. Write a letter to the editor of your local newspaper. Positive, uplifting stories about successful accommodations and working with a disability will help others and bring positive attention to your place of employment. If you are not working and want to work, share your story.

• Mentor others. If you started your nursing career with a disability, write and speak about your experiences. Tell others how you accomplished your goal. Mentor other nurses and nursing students with disabilities. Get involved in a disability organization. There may be a future career path within a disability related organization.

- Adjunct. Opportunities to develop courses taught via the Internet are endless. Try teaching a class for a semester. For Jennifer Krawcheck, RN, teaching nursing was a career path that evolved following a dirt bike accident. She always wanted to teach and didn't let her wheelchair stop her. As one of her nursing students said, "You just ignore her chair like it's not even there because it just doesn't matter" (Helser, 2005). Susan Matt, RN, MN, JD, has a severe hearing loss. She is a Clinical Assistant Professor in the Department of Biobehavioral Nursing and Health Systems at the University of Washington, School of Nursing.

- Research. Conduct research about the experiences of nurses with disabilities. Consider this topic for a master's or doctoral dissertation. Grants are available to support this type of inquiry.

- Get a life outside of nursing. Spend time with family and friends. Participate in sporting activities. Join a Bunko group or book club. Attend plays and cultural activities. Travel. Get a life beyond the walls of your unit.

- Be prepared to relocate to another area. Perhaps a warmer climate, slower pace or a city with good public transportation would be a good move. Think about places you would and would not want to live.

- Stay abreast of national and international disability online networks. Many websites for d/Deaf people post advertisements for employment. Through these networks, there may be people already connected to the local job market in your career field who could provide you with valuable information about the market and possible employment opportunities.

- Conduct a periodic job search and develop self-promotion strategies. Keep your resume or portfolio current. Attend career fairs in your area.

- Start a business. Visit the National Nurses in Business <http://www.nnba.net> to formulate ideas or take a course. Visit The Nurse Entrepreneur Website <http://www.nursefriendly.com/nursing/business.htm> to learn about entrepreneurial opportunities. Susan Nordermo, RN, didn't let vision loss deter her from opening a business called Healing Crossways <http://www.root100.net/hc/about.html>. Susan is a Reiki Master and certified hypnotherapist. She works with clients seeking weight loss, pain control and smoking cessation.

- Keep your spiritual side vibrant. Get or stay involved with a religious or spiritual group. If an organized religion is part of your life, consider becoming a parish nurse in the denomination of your choice, be it at a church, synagogue, temple or mosque.

- Surround yourself with positive people. Nurture positive interpersonal relationships in your work setting. Be as nonconfrontational as possible. Remember the dictum—you can catch more flies with honey than vinegar. Extend small kindnesses to others. Should someone be rude, smile back and show them a better way. This attitude helps make everyone's experience better. Positive attitudes make all the difference in most of life's activities.

◆　　◆　　◆

Adleman, C. S. (2005). Writing your way to health and healing: An interactive workshop [WWW page]. URL www.ExceptionalNurse.com

Adleman, C. S. (2005). Recovering from stroke: A journey toward health [WWW page]. URL www.ExceptionalNurse.com

Cardillo, D. Career alternatives for nurses™ [WWW page]. URL www.dcardillo.com/career_tape.html

Charney, W. & Hudson, A. (2003). *Back injury among healthcare workers.* Boca Raton, FL: CRC Press.

Helser, L. (2005). Spirit isn't broken [WWW page]. URL http://www.azcentral.com/arizonarepublic/northphoenix/articles/1210phx-nurse1210Z3.html#

Holloran, P. (2005). *Walking like a duck: The true story of a nurse walking from addiction to recovery.* Lincoln, NE: iUniverse.

Ritter, R. (2006). *Coping with physical loss and disability.* Ann Arbor, MI: Loving Healing Press.

Serdans, B. (2001). *I'm moving on…are U?*. Philadelphia, PA: Xlibris Corporation.

Zweigle, T.C. (2005). *Psych ward*. Frederick, MD: Publish America.

Conclusion

By Donna Carol Maheady, ARNP, EdD

Nursing with a disability is a challenge, but it is not impossible. The nurses who have shared their stories are living proof of that. A sense of humor, perseverance and a positive attitude helped many of these nurses continue to practice.

Whether you are a student pursuing a nursing degree, a nurse struggling with a disability or a hospital administrator having to accommodate a nurse, creativity is the key to success. There is always another way to accomplish any given task. Find it.

No one knows when a heart attack, stroke or a car accident will leave him or her disabled. But ongoing continuing education, the pursuit of advanced degrees, current certifications, flexibility and an entrepreneurial spirit can help you ensure a bright future, whether or not you ever become disabled.

Nurses with disabilities are entitled to request and receive reasonable accommodation to enable them to perform the essential functions of a job. Furthermore, they have the right to equal enjoyment of the benefits and privileges of employment enjoyed by others. Unfortunately, individuals with disabilities still encounter a great deal of stigma. But by knowing the law, nurses with disabilities can take action to ensure that they are afforded opportunities equal to other nurses.

While it's vital—both for your safety and that of your patients—to know your limitations, it's also important to realize that you may have to work harder than non-disabled colleagues to overcome stereotypes and gain their respect. Don't be afraid to ask for help when you need it, but be willing to lend a hand in return whenever it's needed of you.

Don't give up on a dream because you have become disabled. Find another way to achieve it. Sometimes that means persevering in a current job to prove to your coworkers and hospital administrators that it can be done. Other times, it may mean being more flexible by considering different areas of nursing or finding new ways to use your knowledge outside of direct patient care. Sometimes, a disability can open new doors for you—but only if you are willing to see those possibilities. You may be blinded to them if you only dwell on what you have lost as a result of your condition.

If you need accommodations to be successful in your job, don't be afraid to ask for them. The key is to remember that employers are only obliged to grant reasonable requests. Be prepared to justify your request and explain why it's in the employer's best interest to grant it. Some accommodations can be provided informally and offered simply as helpful gestures from colleagues. When helpful gestures are offered to you, try to return the gesture whenever possible. By making sure your disability is not associated with a difficult working situation for others, you can more readily gain acceptance.

Make sure your employer knows how your disability makes you an especially valuable member of the team. Be your own champion. Keep your eyes open to every possibility along the way. Writing, publishing and bringing positive attention to your place of employment can be helpful. As a nurse, you are used to being an advocate for your patients. Do the same for yourself. Don't be afraid to use assertiveness and nudge things forward. By having the patience and willingness to educate others about how much a person with a disability can accomplish, you can pave the way for other nurses with disabilities as well.

Nurses and administrators need to have greater awareness of the struggles of some of their colleagues to continue practicing. Many nurses are underemployed and long to return to the bedside to engage in direct patient care. Administrators and human resource staffers should facilitate accommodations for more nurses with disabilities. Employment advertisements should state: "Nurses with disabilities *encouraged* to apply." Applicants need to be considered individually, based on their abilities not their limitations. And accommodation plans should be developed that allow essential functions, particularly lifting and CPR, to be achieved in new, creative ways.

Nurses need to reach out to colleagues with disabilities and invite them to stay or come back to work in caring and supportive environments. State nursing boards should examine or re-examine rules and regulations regarding licensure of nurses with disabilities. Additionally, nursing programs need to create more diverse, accommodating academic programs. Nurses and educators need to reach out to students with disabilities, cultivate their passion, harvest the potential and welcome them to the profession.

Nurses need to look at the seat next to them at the nurse's station or in the lounge and move over and make room for a nurse with a disability to find a seat. There is more than enough room for nurses with disabilities within the profession—not just because of the Americans with Disabilities Act, the nursing shortage, litigation or a workers' compensation claim—but simply because it's the right thing to do.

Let's try not to leave any nurse who can work and wants to work behind. The cost to society of underutilizing the hearts and minds of these professionals is staggering.

APPENDIX A

Sample Accommodation Request Letter

The following is an example of what can be included in an accommodation request letter. It is not intended to be legal advice:

Date of Letter
Your name
Your address
Employer's name
Employer's address

Dear (e.g. Supervisor, Manager, Human Resources, Personnel):

Content to consider in body of letter:
- Identify yourself as a person with a disability.
- State that you are requesting accommodations under the ADA (or the Rehabilitation Act of 1973 if you are a federal employee).
- Identify your specific problematic job tasks.
- Identify your accommodation ideas.
- Request your employer's accommodation ideas.
- Refer to attached medical documentation if appropriate.*
- Ask that your employer respond to your request in a reasonable amount of time.

Sincerely,
Your signature

Your printed name
Cc: To appropriate individuals

☛ You may want to attach medical information to your letter to help establish that you are a person with a disability and to document the need for accommodation.

* Source: Department of Labor, Office of Disability Employment Policy, Job Accommodation Network <http://www.jan.wvu.edu>.

Appendix B

Disclosing Your Psychiatric Disability to an Employer

Only you can decide whether and how much to tell your employer about your psychiatric disability. On the positive side, telling your employer about your diagnosis is the only way to protect your legal right to any accommodations you might need to get or keep a job. However, revealing your disability also leaves you open to discrimination, which may limit your opportunities for employment and advancement. It's a complex decision and one you shouldn't make until you've thought it through. Here's what you might want to think about:

Preparing to Disclose

1. Assess your job search skills to determine whether you need help from your therapist or mental health agency to—

   - Initiate contact or arranging an interview with the employer.

   - Interview.

   - Describe your disability.

   - Negotiate the terms of employment.

   - Negotiate accommodations.

2. Identify any potential accommodations you might need during the hiring process or on your first day of work.

3. Explore your feelings about having a mental illness and about sharing that information with others. Remember, no one can force you to disclose if you don't want to.

4. Research potential employers' attitudes toward mental illness and screen out unsupportive employers. Consider—

    - Have they hired someone with a psychiatric disability before?
    - Do they personally know someone with a mental illness?
    - What positive or negative experiences have they had in employing someone with a mental illness?
    - Do they show signs—in newsletters, posted notices, employee education programs about mental illness, etc.—of encouraging a diverse workforce?
    - Do they have a corporate culture that favors flextime, mentoring, telecommuting, flexible benefit plans, and other programs that help employees work efficiently and well?
    - Does the job have certain requirements (e.g., child care or high security) that would put you at a disadvantage if you disclosed your diagnosis?

5. Weigh the benefits and risks of disclosure—

    - Do you need to involve an outside agency to get or keep the job?
    - Do you need accommodation or other employer support?
    - When will you need this accommodation?
    - Do other people in the company need similar accommodation?
    - How stressful will it be for you to hide your disability?

6. If you decide not to disclose, find other ways to get the support you need:

    - Seek out behind-the-scenes support from friends, therapists, etc.
    - Research potential employers who provide this support to all employees.

7. If you decide to disclose, plan in advance how you'll handle it:

    - Who will say it (you, your therapist, your job coach, etc.)?
    - What to say (see below).
    - When to say it.

Under the ADA, a person with a disability can choose to disclose at any time and is not required to disclose at all unless he wants to request an accommodation or wants other protection under the law. Someone with a disability can disclose at any of these times:

- Before the hiring interview.

- During the interview.

- After the interview but before any job offer.

- After a job offer but before starting a job.

- Anytime after beginning a job.

We recommend disclosing sometime before serious problems arise on the job. It is unlikely that you would be protected under the ADA if you disclosed right before you were about to get fired. Employers are most likely to be responsive to a disclosure if they think it is done in good faith and not as a last-ditch effort to keep your job. Who to tell:

- Your supervisor or manager, if he must provide or approve an accommodation.

- The EEO/affirmative action officer or human resources staff, if no immediate accommodation is needed but you would like the protection of the ADA.

- The person interviewing you or human resources staff, if you might need accommodation during the hiring process.

- The employee assistance program staff, if you are already on the job, experiencing difficulties, and need help deciding how, how much, and to whom to disclose.

When You Disclose

1. Decide how specific you will be in describing your psychiatric disability:

    - General terms: a disability, a medical condition or an illness.

    - Vague but more specific terms: a biochemical imbalance, a neurological problem, a brain disorder or difficulty with stress.

    - Specifically referring to mental illness: a mental illness, psychiatric disorder or mental disability.

- Your exact diagnosis: schizophrenia, bipolar disorder, major depression or anxiety disorder.

2. Describe the skills you have that make you able to perform the main duties of the job.

    - Qualifications.

    - Technical skills.

    - General work skills.

3. Describe any functional limitations or behaviors caused by your disability which interfere with your performance (See Steps to Define Functional Limitations).

4. Identify the accommodations you need to overcome those functional limitations or behaviors (See Steps to Identify Reasonable Accommodations).

5. Optional: You may choose to describe the behaviors or symptoms the employer might observe and tell the employer what steps to take as a result.

6. Point the employer to resources for further information:

    - Employment specialist, supported employment provider, rehabilitation counselor or job coach.

    - Doctor or psychiatrist

    - Therapist, counselor or social worker.

    - Job Accommodation Network.

    - ADA Disability and Business Technical Assistance Centers.

    - Others listed in the Resources Section.

7. You may find it helpful to prepare a script to read from. For example:

    - "I have (preferred term for psychiatric disability) that I am recovering from. Currently, I can/have (the skills required) to do (the main duties) of the job, but sometimes (functional limitations) interfere with my ability to (duties you may have trouble performing). It helps if I have (name the specific accommodations you need). I work best when (other accommodations)."

8. You could also add the following information:

   • "Sometimes you might see (symptoms or behaviors associated with symptoms). When you see that, you can (name the action steps for the employer). Here is the number of my (employment specialist, doctor, therapist, previous employer, JAN, etc.) for any information that you might need about my ability to handle the job."

© 1997, 1998 Center for Psychiatric Rehabilitation, Boston University.

APPENDIX C

Dealing with a Difficult Boss

No one is perfect, and everyone is entitled to a bad day now and then. But if you have a difficult boss, you may feel like you have to walk on eggshells every day to prevent problems. The tension of waiting for something to go wrong can sap your belief in your own abilities. Combined with the symptoms of your mental illness, it can make every workday feel like a waking nightmare. Wondering how to deal with a particularly difficult supervisor? Here are some suggestions:

- Meet with a job coach, who can help you determine whether your work style, communication skills, etc., are contributing to the problem. The coach will work with you to improve matters.

- Arrange to meet with your supervisor several times to find out what he expects and needs from you and how you can meet those requirements.

- Keep a detailed written record of any problematic interactions. When did it happen? Where were you at the time? What did your boss say to you? How did you respond? What happened next?

- Don't blow up, slink away or do whatever else you instinctively do when people are angry with you. Losing control makes you look bad, and walking away makes you look like you're challenging your supervisor's authority.

- If you're cursed at, threatened, physically or sexually harassed, or otherwise treated abusively, take your written record of the event to your company's personnel department and your boss's manager.

- If you think your treatment is due to your psychiatric disability, consider filing a complaint under the ADA.

© 1997, 1998 Center for Psychiatric Rehabilitation, Boston University.

Resources

Readers are encouraged to explore the World Wide Web for disability-specific organizations. The scope of the following list is general and not meant to be all-inclusive.

Education and Career Information

American Nurses Association: www.ana.org

National League for Nursing: www.nln.org

The National League for Nursing Accrediting Commission: www.nlnac.org/home.htm

National Council of State Boards of Nursing: www.ncsbn.org

University of Salford School of Nursing Program for Deaf Students: www.nursing.salford.ac.uk/pioneers.html

Nurses with Disabilities

ExceptionalNurse.com: www.ExceptionalNurse.com

Healthcare Professionals with a Disability in the United Kingdom: www.david-j-wright.staff.shef.ac.uk/HCP-disability/

The Center for Disabilities in the Health Professions: www.westernu.edu/xp/edu/cdihp/about.xml

HIV Positive Health Care Professionals: www.positivehealthcareprofessionals.com

Association of Nurses in AIDS Care: www.anacnet.org

Work Injured Nurses' Group: www.wingusa.org

Reasonable Accommodations/Legal Resources

The ADA and Information Technology Assistance Center:
www.adata.org

Office of the Americans with Disabilities Act
Civil Rights Division, U.S. Department of Justice
www.usdoj.gov/crt/ada/adahom1.htm

The U.S. Equal Employment Opportunity Commission:
www.eeoc.gov/policy/guidance.html

Telework as a Reasonable Accommodation:
www.eeoc.gov./facts/telework.html

Job Accommodation Network: www.jan.wvu.edu/soar

Guide Dogs/Service Animals: www.usdoj.gov/crt/ada/animal.htm

Family Medical Leave: www.dol.gov/esa/whd/fmla

Discussion Groups

Is There a Place in Nursing for RNs/LPNs Who Are Disabled?
www.medscape.com/nurses-home

Nurses with dystonia and other disabilities:
www.care4dystonia.org/messageboards.htm

Newsletter

The Exceptional Nurse Newsletter: www.ExceptionalNurse.com

Mental Health Issues

Boston University Center for Psychiatric Rehabilitation:
www.bu.edu/cpr/reasaccom

U.S. Department of Health and Human Services,
Substance Abuse and Mental Health Services Administration:
http://stopstigma.samhsa.gov

The Carter Center: www.cartercenter.org/healthprograms/591_adoc6.htm

Nurses with Hearing Loss

Association of Medical Professionals with Hearing Loss:
www.AMPHL.org

Northeast Technical Assistance Center: www.netac.rit.edu/about.html

PEPNet.org: www.PepNet.org.

Promoting Awareness in Healthcare, Medical and Deaf:
www.urmc.rochester.edu/smd/stdnt/pahmd/welcome.htm

Self Help for Hard of Hearing People, Inc.: www.shhh.org

UK Health Professionals with Hearing Loss: www.hphl.org.uk

Nurses in Recovery

INA: International Nurses Anonymous: www.intnursesanon.org

Nurses in Recovery: www.brucienne.com/nir

Workplace Violence

International Council of Nurses: www.icn.ch

Listening Devices

Beyond Hearing Aids: www.beyondhearingaids.com

Phonic Ear: www.phonicear.com

Reading Aid

Reading Pen Portable Assistive Reading Device:
www.wizcomtech.com/Wizcom/products/products.asp?fid=78

Financial Information/Resources/Assistance

Internal Revenue Service
Tax Highlights for Persons with Disabilities
www.irs.gov

Social Security Administration
U.S. Department of Health and Human Services
www.ssa.gov

Nurseshouse.org: www.Nurseshouse.org

Scholarships: www.ExceptionalNurse.com

Rehabilitation Services

Department of Vocational Rehabilitation (VR)
Vocational Rehabilitation is a nationwide federal-state program for assisting eligible people with disabilities. The VR program is an eligibility program, rather than an entitlement program. Agency titles vary. Contact a state education agency, public library, or the Governor's Committee on Employment of People with Disabilities to get contact information for your local VR agency. VR provides support services needed to prepare people with disabilities for work.

Social Security Online:
www.ssa.gov/work/serviceproviders/rehabproviders.html

Department off Veterans Affairs
Vocational Rehabilitation and Counseling Programs
www.vba.va.gov/bln/vre/vreindex.htm

Educational Resources

Captioned Media Program
National Association of the Deaf
www.cfv.org

Library Reproduction Service: www.LRS-LARGEPRINT.com

National Library Service for the Blind and Physically Handicapped
Library of Congress
www.loc.gov/nls

Recording for the Blind and Dyslexic, Inc.: www.rfbd.org

Disabilities, Opportunities, Internetworking and Technology:
www.washington.edu/doit/Faculty

Equipment

Stethoscopes.com: www.stethoscopes.com

Welch Allyn: www.welchallyn.com

Allheart.com: www.allheart.com

Ultrascopes.com: www.ultrascopes.com

Cardionics Inc.: www.cardionics.com

One-Hand Blood Pressure Monitors: www.stethoscopes.com

Vision Loss

Sight Connection: www.sightconnection.com

Independent Living: www.independentliving.com

Standing Wheelchairs

Levo USA: www.levousa.com/E/Organis/levoag.htm

See-Through Surgical Mask Availability

The Association of Medical Professionals with Hearing Loss:
www.AMPHL.org

Examination Tables

Hausmann Powermatic Wheelchair Accessible Power Table:
www.hausmann.com/medmain.html

Computers

IBM Accessibility Center: www.ibm.com/able

Mouse adapter:
http://domino.research.ibm.com/comm/pr.nsf/pages/
news.20050314_mouseadapter.html

Apple Computers: www.apple.com/disability

Microsoft: www.microsoft.com/enable/default.aspx

Business

National Nurses in Business Association: www.nnba.net

References

Bain, E., Kunz, M., & Maheady, D. (2005). Question & answer. Working with disability [WWW page]. URL http://nursing.advanceweb.com/common/ EditorialSearch/AViewer.aspx?AN= NW_05oct10_n2p12.html&AD=10-10-2005

Creamer, B. (2003). Wheelchair fails to deter paraplegic from nurse's life [WWW page]. URL http://the.honoluluadvertiser.com/article/2003/Dec/ 28/ln/ln10a.html

Dresen, B. (2005). The other side of the bed. *Advance for LPNs, 5* (7), 7A.

Dunbar, C. (2005). Stories of hope and joy. Nursing spectrum [WWW page]. URL http://community.nursingspectrum. com/MagazineArticles/article.cfm?AID=18882

Fleming, S., & Maheady, D. (2004). Empowering persons with disabilities. *AWHONN lifelines, 8* (6), 534-537.

Jackson-Ferguson, W.M. (2005). Help or hinder? [WWW page]. URL http:// nursing.advanceweb.com/common/EditorialSearch/ AViewer.aspx?CC=60336

Koviack, P. (2004). A review of the effect of an accommodation program to support nurses with functional limitations. *Nursing economics, 22* (6) (5), 320-324, 355.

Loy, B. (2006). Accommodations, ADA and light duty. Consultants' Corner. Job Accommodations Network, Office of Disability Employment Policy, U.S. Department of Labor. [WWW page]. URL http://www.jan.wvu. edu/corner/index.htm

Maheady, D.C., Fleming, S. (2005, Summer). Nursing with the hand you are given. *Minority nurse*, 50-54.

Maheady, D.C., Fleming, S. (2005, Spring). Homework for future nursing students with disabilities. *Minority nurse,* 60-64

Maheady, D. C. (2005). Teaching nursing students with disabilities. In L. Caputi (Ed.), *Teaching nursing: The art and science: Volume 3.* Glen Ellyn, IL: College of DuPage Press.

Maheady, D. (2004). Positions wanted: Nurses with disabilities. *American journal of nursing, 104* (3), 13.

Maheady, D. (2004). Planning for success [WWW page]. URL http://www.nursingspectrum.com/StudentsCorner/StudentFeatures/PlanningForSuccess_stk.htm

Maheady, D. (2003). *Nursing students with disabilities change the course.* River Edge, NJ: Exceptional Parent Press.

Maheady, D. (1999). Jumping through hoops, walking on eggshells: The experiences of nursing students with disabilities. *Journal of nursing education, 38* (4), 162-170.

Matt, S.B., & Butterfield, P. (2006). Changing the disability climate: promoting tolerance in the workplace. *AAOHN Journal, 54 (3), 129-133.*

Medical News Today (2005). Blind woman will pursue her dream of becoming a nurse [WWW page]. URL http://www.medicalnewstoday.com/medicalnews.php?newsid=19122

Miller, K. (2005). Medical College of Georgia nursing student overcomes obstacles to pursue degree [WWW page]. URL http://www.mcg.edu/news/2005NewsRel/KSTrapp111805.html

Morris, R. (2003). Cope with Scopes. Stethoscopes and Hearing Aids-What are the options? [WWW page]. URL http://www.healthyhearing.com/library/article_content.asp?article_id=197

Nettina, S. (2003). The untapped nursing workpool: Nurses with disabilities [WWW page]. URL http://www.medscape.com/viewarticle/452605_1

Rennert, N., Morris, B., and Barrere, C.C. (2004, February). How to cope with scopes: Stethoscope selection and use with hearing aids and CIs. [WWW

page]. URL http://www.hearingreview.com/Articles.
ASP?articleid=H0402F04

Restifo, V. (2001). Tips for disabled nurses [WWW page]. URL http://
community.nursingspectrum.com/MagazineArticles/arti-
cle.cfm?AID=3399

Rose, J.F. (2005). Disabled nurses: Disclosure and safe practice [WWW page].
URL http://www.nursezone.com/Stories/SpotlightOnNurses.
asp?articleID=13386

Rosenberg, H. (2005). Against all odds: Paraplegic nurse welcomed back to work
at the Bronx Division of Jewish Home and Hospital Lifecare System.
Advance for nurses, 5 (22), 15.

Scally, R. (2003). Disabilities can't stop these nurses [WWW page]. URL http://
www.nursezone.com/stories/SpotlightOnNurses.asp?articleID=10861

Yox, S. (2003). Do we support nurse colleagues who have disabilities? [WWW
page]. URL http://www.medscape.com/viewarticle/449392

Readers are invited to visit www.ExceptionalNurse.com for additional information and to subscribe to the ExceptionalNurse.com newsletter.

About the Author

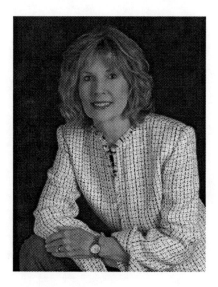

Donna Carol Maheady, ARNP, EdD, the mother of a daughter with disabilities, is a Pediatric Nurse Practitioner and Adjunct Assistant Professor in the Christine E. Lynn College of Nursing at Florida Atlantic University. Dr. Maheady is the author of *Nursing Students with Disabilities Change the Course* and the founder of www.ExceptionalNurse.com.

978-0-595-39649-8
0-595-39649-6

Printed in the United States
71344LV00004B/361-363